Statistics for Biology and Health

Series Editors
K. Dietz, M. Gail, K. Krickeberg, J. Samet, A. Tsiatis

Springer

New York
Berlin
Heidelberg
Hong Kong
London
Milan
Paris
Tokyo

Statistics for Biology and Health

Borchers/Buckland/Zucchini: Estimating Animal Abundance: Closed Populations.

Everitt/Rabe-Hesketh: Analyzing Medical Data Using S-PLUS.

Ewens/Grant: Statistical Methods in Bioinformatics: An Introduction.

Hougaard: Analysis of Multivariate Survival Data.

Klein/Moeschberger: Survival Analysis: Techniques for Censored and Truncated Data, 2nd ed.

Kleinbaum: Survival Analysis: A Self-Learning Text.

Kleinbaum/Klein: Logistic Regression: A Self-Learning Text, 2nd ed.

Lange: Mathematical and Statistical Methods for Genetic Analysis, 2nd ed.

Manton/Singer/Suzman: Forecasting the Health of Elderly Populations.

Moyé: Multiple Analyses in Clinical Trials: Fundamentals for Investigators.

Parmigiani/Garrett/Irizarry/Zeger: The Analysis of Gene Expression Data: Methods and Software.

Salsburg: The Use of Restricted Significance Tests in Clinical Trials.

Simon/Korn/McShane/Radmacher/Wright/Zhao: Design and Analysis of DNA Microarray Investigations.

Sorensen/Gianola: Likelihood, Bayesian, and MCMC Methods in Quantitative Genetics.

Therneau/Grambsch: Modeling Survival Data: Extending the Cox Model.

Zhang/Singer: Recursive Partitioning in the Health Sciences.

Richard M. Simon   Edward L. Korn
Lisa M. McShane   Michael D. Radmacher
George W. Wright   Yingdong Zhao

Design and Analysis of DNA Microarray Investigations

With 58 Figures, 15 in Full color

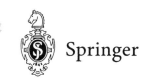

Springer

Richard M. Simon
Edward L. Korn
Lisa M. McShane
George W. Wright
Yingdong Zhao
Biometric Research Branch
National Cancer Institute
9000 Rockville Pike
MSC 7434
Bethesda, MD 20892-7434

Michael D. Radmacher
Departments of Mathematics
  & Biology
Kenyon College
Gambier, OH 43022

Series Editors
K. Dietz
Institut für Medizinische Biometrie
Universität Tübingen
Westbahnhofstrasse 55
D-72070 Tübingen
Germany

M. Gail
National Cancer Institute
Rockville, MD 20892
USA

K. Krickeberg
Le Chatelet
F-63270 Manglieu
France

J. Samet
Department of Epidemiology
School of Public Health
Johns Hopkins University
615 Wolfe Street
Baltimore, MD 21205-2103
USA

A. Tsiatis
Department of Statistics
North Carolina State University
Raleigh, NC 27695
USA

Library of Congress Cataloging-in-Publication Data
Design and analysis of DNA microarray investigations / Richard M. Simon . . . [et al.].
    p. cm. — (Statistics for biology and health)
    ISBN 0-387-00135-2 (hbk. : alk. paper)
    1. DNA microarrays—Statistical methods.   I. Simon, Richard M., 1943–   II. Series.
   QP624.5.D726D475 2003
   572.8'65—dc21   2003054790

ISBN 0-387-00135-2   Printed on acid-free paper.

Printed in the United States of America.

9 8 7 6 5 4 3 2 1   SPIN 10898178

www.springer-ny.com

Springer-Verlag New York Berlin Heidelberg
A member of BertelsmannSpringer Science+Business Media GmbH

Acknowledgments

We thank our colleagues at the National Cancer Institute who have given us the opportunity to become involved in cancer genomics, and to contribute to discovery of a new generation of therapeutics based on improved knowledge of tumor biology. We particularly thank Dr. Robert Wittes for supporting the establishment of the Molecular Statistics and Bioinformatics Section of the Biometric Research Branch and providing it with the independence to develop expertise, conduct independent research, and establish a unique multidisciplinary environment in which methodologists and experimentalists can interact.

We thank Amy Peng Lam for her development of BRB-ArrayTools in collaboration with Richard Simon, and for her many contributions to our microarray analyses. Thanks to Dr. Ming-Chung Li for excellent statistical computing support, to Dr. James P. Brody for permission to use Figure 3.1, to the National Human Genome Research Institute for illustrations 2.1 and A.1–A.5 from their Talking Glossary website, to Drs. Tatiana Dracheva, Jin Jen, and Joanna Shih for providing Affymetrix GeneChip^{TM} images, to Mr. Erik Marchese at Affymetrix for technical consultation, and to Dr. Laura Lee Johnson for a careful reading of an earlier draft.

Richard M. Simon
Edward L. Korn
Lisa M. McShane
Michael D. Radmacher
George W. Wright
Yingdong Zhao
Bethesda, MD

Contents

1

Introduction

DNA microarrays are an important technology for studying gene expression. With a single hybridization, the level of expression of thousands of genes, or even an entire genome, can be estimated for a sample of cells. Consequently, many laboratories are attempting to utilize DNA microarrays in their research. Whereas laboratories are well prepared to address the significant experimental challenges in obtaining reproducible data from this RNA-based assay, investigators are less prepared to analyze the large volumes of data produced by DNA microarrays.

Although many software packages have been developed for the analysis of DNA microarray data, software alone is insufficient. One needs knowledge about the various aspects of data analysis in order to select and utilize software effectively. There is a plethora of analysis methods being published and it is difficult for biologists to determine which methods are valid and appropriate for their problems.

Many scientists have learned that software is not an adequate substitute for biostatistical knowledge and seek statistical collaborators. Unfortunately, there is presently a shortage of statisticians who are available and knowledgeable about DNA microarrays. For statisticians to be effective collaborators in any area, they must invest the time to understand the subject matter area and become familiar with the literature so that they can ask the right questions and identify the key issues.

Our objectives in this book are twofold: to provide scientists with information about the design and analysis of studies using DNA microarrays that will enable them to plan and analyze their own studies or to work with statistical collaborators effectively, and to aid statistical and computational scientists wishing to develop expertise in this area.

We believe that the design and analysis of microarray studies should be driven by the objectives of the experiment. We have identified several common types of objectives and for each type we have presented methods that we believe are statistically sound and effective. These methods are described in a manner that we believe will be understandable to most scientists. We emphasize the concepts behind the methods rather than the mechanics of the use of the formulas. In most cases, the methods are available in existing software and the investigator will need knowledge of concepts to select methods and software more than knowledge of formulas for doing the calculations by hand. We have made the data used as examples in this book available on our Web site (see Appendix B) and have provided readers with a tutorial on the use of our BRB-ArrayTools software for analysis of these datasets. BRB-ArrayTools, described in Appendix C, is a menu-driven program incorporating many advanced analysis features but easily usable by scientists. BRB-ArrayTools is available without charge for noncommercial purposes.

We have tried to keep each chapter focused and relatively short in order to enhance its readability. Analytic methods for DNA microarray data are an active area of research. We have presented specific methods that we have found to be valid and useful. Although we generally describe a variety of approaches to analysis, we have not tried to be encyclopedic with regard to the literature. We hope that this serves the needs of most scientists looking for expert advice about sound and effective methods and also the needs of statistical and computational scientists looking for a broader coverage of the literature. Most of the material included has been written to be understandable to biological scientists without substantial statistical training. We have avoided mathematical and statistical derivations and nonessential notation.

Chapter 2 is a brief description of microarray platforms commonly used for gene expression profiling, including dual-label cDNA and oligonucleotide platforms and Affymetrix GeneChip^{TM} arrays. Some experimentalists may choose to skip this chapter. Although microarrays can also be used for purposes other than gene expression profiling, such as sequencing and genotyping, these latter applications are not the focus of this book.

Chapter 3 discusses important aspects of the design of studies that use DNA microarrays. A complete presentation of the area of biomedical study design is not possible in one chapter, but we attempt to address many topics of special relevance in DNA microarray based studies.

Chapter 4 addresses the creation and analysis of images of intensities on microarrays after hybridization of labeled targets to the immobilized probes. That is, we discuss how pixel-level data are converted to probe-level or gene-level summaries. Although scientists generally do not do their own image analysis, some need to select software and to evaluate their images. Hence a basic understanding of the issues involved is useful.

Chapters 5 and 6 examine a variety of signal-processing issues, which must be addressed before the objective-directed analysis strategy is implemented. Chapter 5 covers methods of evaluating quality of microarray data. These issues are discussed separately for dual-label arrays and for GeneChips^{TM}. Chapter 6 addresses issues of normalization. Normalization is necessary because the raw intensities of labeled targets vary among arrays due to sources of experimental variability independent of level of expression. The objectives of normalization are somewhat different for dual-label arrays and for GeneChips^{TM}, and both are discussed.

Chapters 7 through 9 present analysis strategies for studies where the major objectives are class comparison, class prediction, and class discovery, respectively. In class comparison problems discussed in Chapter 7 there is a predefined classification of the specimens and the objective is usually to determine which genes are differentially expressed among the classes. For example, comparing expression profiles for different types of tissue or for the same tissue under different conditions are class comparison objectives.

In some studies, particularly those involving expression profiles of diseased human tissues, there are predefined classes and the emphasis is on attempting to develop a gene expression-based predictor of the class to which a new specimen belongs. Such class prediction problems, and the related problem of prognostic prediction, are addressed in Chapter 8. For example, we may have tissues from patients with a specified disease who have received a specific treatment. One class may be those specimens from patients who responded to the treatment and the other class may be those tissues from patients who did not respond. The objective may be to predict whether a new patient is likely to respond based on the expression profile of his or her tissue specimen. Accurate prediction is of obvious value in treatment selection. In Chapter 8 we discuss the key components of a class prediction algorithm and describe several commonly used methods of prediction.

Chapter 9 addresses class discovery objectives. This includes discovery of new groupings or taxonomies of the specimens, based on expression profiles. Discovering classes of coexpressed and potentially coregulated genes is also a discovery objective. Class discovery is usually adressed using methods of cluster analysis. Chapter 9 also describes principal components analysis and multidimensional scaling and the graphical displays associated with these methods.

We present the material in Chapters 7 through 9 in a relatively nonmathematical style that will be understandable to a broad range of scientists and to illustrate many of the methods with examples.

Appendix A provides basic information on the biology of gene expression for statistical and computational scientists who do not have biological training. Appendix B provides information about the gene expression datasets that are used as examples in this book. Learning about analysis of DNA microarray data is facilitated by experience analyzing real data. Therefore, on our Web site http://linus.nci.nih.gov/~brb we provide the datasets used as examples in this book. Individuals can practice analyzing these datasets, or their own data, using the software of their choice. Appendix C describes the BRB-ArrayTools software. This software includes many of the methods described in the text and is regularly being extended with more tools based upon our experience in the analysis of microarray data. Again, BRB-ArrayTools is available on our Web site without charge for noncommercial purposes. It can be licensed from the National Institutes of Health by commercial organizations.

2

DNA Microarray Technology

2.1 Overview

DNA microarrays are assays for quantifying the types and amounts of mRNA transcripts present in a collection of cells. The number of mRNA molecules derived from transcription of a given gene is an approximate estimate of the level of expression of that gene; see Appendix A for basic information on the biology of gene expression. RNA is extracted from the specimen and the mRNA is isolated. The mRNA transcripts are then converted to a form of labeled polynucleotides, called targets, and placed on the microarray. Details of the labeling process are provided later in this chapter.

The microarray consists of a solid surface on which strands of polynucleotides have been attached in specified positions. We refer to the polynucleotides immobilized on the solid surface as *probes*. The probes consist either of cDNA printed on the surface or shorter *oligonucleotides* synthesized or deposited on the surface. The labeled targets bind by hybridization to the probes on the array with which they share sufficient sequence complementarity. After allowing sufficient time for the hybridization reaction, the excess sample is washed off the solid surface. At that point, each probe on the microarray should be bound to a quantity of labeled target that is proportional to the level of expression of the gene represented by that probe. By measuring the intensity of label bound to each probe, one obtains numbers that, after adjustment for technical artifacts, should provide an estimate of the level of expression of all the corresponding genes.

2.2 Measuring Label Intensity

The amount of labeled target bound to each polynucleotide probe is quantified by illuminating the solid surface with laser light of a frequency tuned to the fluorescent label employed, and then measuring the intensity of fluorescence over each probe on the array. This intensity of fluorescence should be proportional to the number of molecules of target bound to the probe. For a given number of bound molecules, other factors that can influence the intensity of fluorescence include the labeling efficiency, the number of polynucleotide strands in the probe, the laser voltage, and the photomultiplier tube setting. The number of bound molecules will be affected by the number of cells in the specimen, the RNA extraction efficiency, and the spatial distribution of labeled sample on the array.

The fluorescence emitted by molecules of targets bound to a probe is measured by a detector. Most commercial scanners use confocal microscopy detection. A confocal microscope focuses the photons originating in a very small region on the array to a photomultiplier tube. By collecting photons from one very small region at a time, the confocal method is effective in limiting contamination of the signal by other sources of fluorescence. This is important because the fluorescent signal emitted by the fluorophore is relatively weak. The resolution of most commercial confocal microscope-based scanners is about 3 μm, much less than the diameter of the region containing the probe. The array is scanned, collecting photons from each 3 μm region (pixel). At each step of the scan, the photons are focused into a photomultiplier tube where the photon density is translated into an electrical current which is amplified and digitized. If there are two samples cohybridized to the array with two fluorophores, the array is scanned for each label. With many systems, the array is scanned twice for each label and the average intensities recorded.

The fluorescent microscope does not directly measure the intensity of fluorescence over each probe. The instrument does not even know where the probes are located on the surface of the array. Instead, the microscope measures the intensity of fluorescence at each location of an imaginary grid covering the array surface. The grid locations are called *pixels*, short for picture elements. The distance between pixels is much less than the distance between probes. The output of the fluorescent microscope is a computer file, called an *image file*, giving the intensity of fluorescence measurement at each pixel. If two labeled samples were cohybridized, then two files are output, one corresponding to each label, or each *channel*. An image analysis algorithm processes these image files to estimate the intensity of label in each channel over each probe on the array, as described in Chapter 4.

2.3 Labeling Methods

For glass slide arrays the mRNA is usually reverse-transcribed to complementary DNA (cDNA), and a fluorescent label is incorporated into the cDNA during or after the reverse transcription reaction. The labeled cDNA is then placed on the microarray.

For Affymetrix GeneChip™ arrays the preparation of labeled targets is somewhat different (Affymetrix 2000). After isolation of mRNA, cDNA is synthesized. The cDNA is used as a template for T7 RNA polymerase to amplify the cDNA into synthesized cRNA molecules. In this amplification step a biotin label is introduced into the cRNA. The cRNA molecules are then fragmented into molecules 80 to100 nucleotides long. The biotin-labeled cRNA fragments are then hybridized to the GeneChip^{TM}. After hybridization, the bound cRNA fragments are stained with a biotin antibody.

2.4 Printed Microarrays

Microarrays differ in many important details. cDNA microarrays usually consist of probes of cDNA robotically printed on a microscope slide coated with poly-lysine or poly-amine to enhance absorption of the DNA probes (Schena et al. 1995, 2000). The robotic printers have several pins arranged in a rectangular pattern (Figure 2.1). For example, if there are four pins, then for

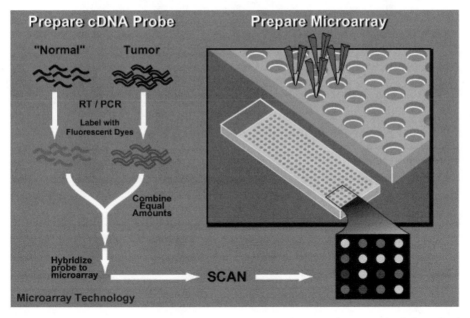

Fig. 2.1. Schematic of robotic printing of spots for cDNA array (right) and of processing of RNA samples for cohybridization to array.

each location of the robotic arm, four spots will be printed. At any time, the pins are loaded with cDNA from four different inventory wells and these PCR product clones are printed on each array of the print run. Then the pins are automatically washed and loaded with four other clones. The arm advances either horizontally or vertically an amount equal to the distance between spots, and the four clones are printed on all of the arrays of the print run. Thus, for a four-pin printer, the spots on the array are printed in four rectangular grids corresponding to the rectangular arrangement of the robotic pins (Figure 2.2). The spots of each grid are printed with the same pin of the robot. The distance between the spots corresponds to the distance that the robotic arm moves between loadings of the pins, and the distance between the grids corresponds to the distance between the pins.

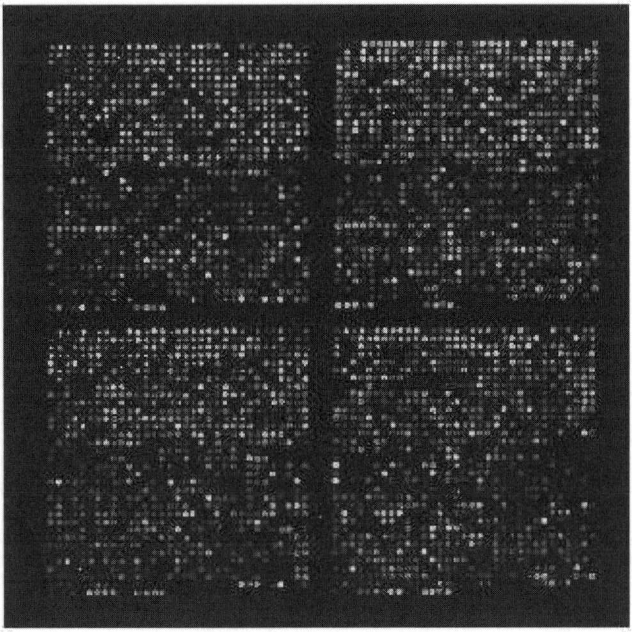

Fig. 2.2. A typical cDNA microarray image with two rows and two columns of grids.

Because the cDNA probes are generally several hundred bases long, stringent hybridization conditions can be employed and cross-reactivity is limited. However, robotic printing often results in substantial variability in the size and shape of corresponding spots on different arrays. Also, with cDNA arrays, the labeled sample is not uniformly distributed across the face of the array and the distribution of the sample differs among otherwise identical arrays. Hence direct comparison of intensities of corresponding probes on different arrays is problematic. Some of the interarray variability can be eliminated by a statistical "normalization" described in Chapter 4. Even after normalization, however, there is often substantial variability among corresponding spots on different arrays. Much of this variability can be controlled by co-hybridizing two samples on the same array. The two cDNA samples are labeled with different fluorescent dyes. By using two laser sources, the intensity of fluorescence in each of the two frequency channels is measured over each probe. The second sample may represent either a specimen whose expression profile relative to the first specimen is of biological interest, or a reference sample used on all arrays in order to control experimental variability.

Externally synthesized oligonucleotides can also be robotically printed on coated glass slides. Because sample distribution across the face of the arrays remains variable, much of the interslide variability that is characteristic of cDNA arrays also applies to printed oligonucleotide arrays. Consequently, co-hybridization of two separately labeled samples is also advantageous.

2.5 Affymetrix GeneChip^{TM} Arrays

Affymetrix GeneChip^{TM} arrays have oligonucleotide probes lithographically synthesized directly on the array. The array in this case is not a glass slide, but a silicon chip (Fodor et al. 1991). The oligonucleotides at all locations on the chip are synthesized in parallel. At the first step, the chip is bathed in a solution containing a precursor to one of the four nucleotides, say G. The synthesis of a nucleotide and attachment of the nucleotide to the anchor or the partially constructed oligonucleotide chain is light actuated. A mask is employed to ensure that light reaches only those addresses where the next nucleotide in the desired sequence is that represented by the current bath, say G. The in situ synthesis continues in this manner with multiple baths, washes, and masks employed.

The probes on GeneChip^{TM} arrays are more homogeneous and less variable relative to cDNA arrays. Inter array variability due to sample distribution effects is also minimized because the samples are circulated inside the GeneChip^{TM} during hybridization. Because of these reductions in inter array variability, a single sample is usually hybridized to GeneChips^{TM}.

The expense of fabrication and frequency of sequence errors for Gene-Chips^{TM} increase with the length of the oligonucleotide probes employed, therefore relatively short 25 mer oligonucleotides are generally used. In order to obtain sufficient binding strength from 25 mer oligonucleotides, the hybridization conditions must be made less stringent than for cDNA arrays or longer spotted oligonucleotide arrays. Consequently, substantial cross hybridization is possible.

Affymetrix attempts to deal with the cross-hybridization problem by using multiple *probe pairs* for each target transcript (Lockhart et al. 1996). A probe pair consists of a 25 mer oligonucleotide perfectly complementary to a 25 nucleotide sequence of an exon of the target gene, and a 25 mer that differs from that perfect match probe by a single mismatched nucleotide at the central position. Affymetrix expects that the mismatched probe should not hybridize well to the target transcript but should hybridize to many transcripts to which the perfect-match oligonucleotide cross-hybridizes. Thus the intensity of signal at the perfect match probe minus the intensity at the mismatched paired probe may be a better estimate of the intensity due to hybridization to the true target transcript.

Current GeneChips^{TM} use 11 to16 probe pairs for each target gene but the lengths of the probes are smaller than for cDNA arrays. The differences in perfect-match minus mismatch intensities are averaged across the probe pairs to give an estimate of intensity of hybridization to the target transcript; see Section 4.3.

2.6 Other Microarray Platforms

Several companies such as Protogene (Menlo Park, CA) and Agilent Technologies (Palo Alto, CA) in collaboration with Rosetta Inpharmatics (Kirkland, WA) have developed methods of in situ synthesis of oligonucleotides on glass arrays using ink-jet technology that does not require photolithography. The ink-jet technology of Agilent can also be used to attach pre synthesized DNA probes to glass slides.

Another class of DNA microarrays utilizes cDNA probes printed on a nylon membrane, and radioactive labeling of the sample. The radioactive label provides a stronger signal than fluorescent dye. This is useful when the amount of mRNA available for labeling is limited, but the wide scattering of label limits the density of probes that can be printed on the array, and larger format arrays are necessary. Although most of the principles of experimental design and analysis apply equally to arrays using radioactively labeled samples as to arrays using fluorescent labels, we generally talk in terms of the latter.

3

Design of DNA Microarray Experiments

3.1 Introduction

Microarray based experiments, like all experiments, should be carefully planned. Careful planning begins with a clear objective. The objective drives the selection of specimens and the specification of an appropriate analysis strategy. It is a common misconception that microarray experiments do not require planning or objectives; in this view, expression profiles are placed in a pattern recognition blackbox and discoveries emerge. Although pattern recognition algorithms have a role for some objectives involving microarrays, most successful microarray-based experiments have a definite focus.

There is substantial confusion about the role of "hypothesis testing" in studies using microarrays. It is true that microarray-based research is generally not based on a mechanistic biological hypothesis focused on specific genes. Other technologies are more suitable for testing hypotheses about specific genes. Nevertheless, most good microarray experiments are based on a hypothesis. For example, the hypothesis might be that there are genes whose expression is up-regulated or down-regulated in a tumor compared to normal tissue of the same tissue type. Or, the hypothesis might be that different tumors of the same tissue type and the same stage are not homogeneous with regard to gene expression profiles. Clearly identifying the general hypothesis of the study is important for ensuring that the type and number of specimens collected are appropriate. Clarity on the general hypotheses is also important for selecting methods of data analysis. A DNA microarray is just a highly parallel assay. It does not herald an era in which good practices of carefully thinking about the objectives of the experiment and of carefully planning the experiment and its analysis are obsolete.

Because DNA microarray investigations are not focused on a prespecified gene-specific hypothesis, there is much more opportunity for spurious findings than with more traditional types of investigations. Although the contexts in which microarrays are used are exploratory, strong claims are often made about which genes are differentially expressed under specified conditions, which are disregulated in diseased tissue, and which are predictive of response to treatment. The serious multiplicity problems inherent in examining expression profiles of tens of thousands of genes mandate careful planning and special forms of analysis in order to avoid being swamped by spurious associations.

Design issues can be divided into those relating to the design of the DNA microarray assay itself and issues involving the selection, labeling, and arraying of the specimens to be assayed. In this chapter, we focus on the latter issues. Section 3.2 describes the importance of defining the study objectives for designing a microarray study. Section 3.3 discusses the difficulties in satisfying study objectives when only two RNA samples are compared. The sources of variation and the levels of replication of the experiment, discussed in Section 3.4, are important to consider when designing a study. Section 3.5 discusses the possibility of pooling samples and assaying the pooled sample with a microarray. With dual-label microarrays, the different ways of pairing and labeling the samples are discussed in Sections 3.6 and 3.7, respectively. The chapter ends with a discussion of the sample sizes required to meet the study objectives.

3.2 Study Objectives

DNA microarrays are useful in a wide variety of investigations with a wide variety of objectives. Many of these objectives fall into the following categories.

3.2.1 Class Comparison

Class comparison focuses on determining whether gene expression profiles differ among samples selected from predefined classes and identifying which genes are differentially expressed among the classes. For example, the classes may represent different tissue types, the same tissue under different experimental conditions, or the same tissue type for different classes of individuals. In cancer studies, the classes often represent distinct categories of tumors differing with regard to stage, primary site, genetic mutations present, or with regard to response to therapy; the specimens may represent tissue taken before or after treatment or experimental intervention. There are many study objectives that can be identified as class comparison. The defining characteristic of class comparison is that the classes are predefined independently of the expression profiles. Many studies are performed to compare gene expression for several types of class definition. For example, two genotypes of mice may be studied under two different experimental conditions. One analysis may address differences in gene expression for the two types of animals under the same experimental condition and the other analysis may address the effect of the experimental intervention on gene expression for a given genotype.

3.2.2 Class Prediction

Class prediction is similar to class comparison except that the emphasis is on developing a statistical model that can predict to which class a new specimen belongs based on its expression profile. This usually requires identifying which genes are informative for distinguishing the predefined classes, using these genes to develop a statistical prediction model, and estimating the accuracy of the predictor. Class prediction is important for medical problems of diagnostic classification, prognostic prediction, and treatment selection.

3.2.3 Class Discovery

Another type of microarray study involves the identification of novel sub-types of specimens within a population. This objective is based on the idea that important biological differences among specimens that are clinically and morphologically similar may be discernible at the molecular level. For example, many microarray studies in cancer have the objective of developing a taxonomy of cancers that originate in a given organ site in order to identify subclasses of tumors that are biologically homogeneous and whose expression profiles either reflect different cells of origin or other differences in disease pathogenesis (Alizadeh et al. 2000; Bittner et al. 2000). These studies may uncover biological features of the disease that pave the way for development of improved treatments by identification of molecular targets for therapy.

3.2.4 Pathway Analysis

The objective of some studies is the identification of genes that are coregulated or which occur in the same biochemical pathway. One widely noted example is the identification of cell cycle genes in yeast (Spellman et al. 1998). Pathway analysis is often based on performing an experimental intervention and comparing expression profiles of specimens collected before and at various time intervals after the experimental intervention. In some cases, however, pathway analysis may involve comparing the wild type organism to genetically altered variants.

3.3 Comparing Two RNA Samples

The initial cDNA microarray studies involved the cohybridization of one mRNA sample labeled with one fluorescent dye and a second mRNA sample labeled with a second fluorescent dye on a single microarray (DeRisi et al. 1996). This type of study, and the high cost of microarrays, left many investigators hoping and believing that no replication was needed. It also led to the publication of a variety of statistical methods for comparing the expression levels in the two channels at each gene on a single microarray. Even today,

Affymetrix software is designed to compare gene expression on just two arrays (one sample on each array) and to compare two classes of specimens one must compare the specimens two at a time (Affymetrix 2002).

The main problems with drawing conclusions based on comparing two RNA samples apply to both dual-label and Affymetrix arrays. First, the relative intensity for a given gene in the two specimens can reflect an experimental artifact in tissue handling, cell culture conditions, RNA extraction, labeling, or hybridization to the arrays that is not removed by the normalization process. The analysis of two RNA samples each arrayed once provides very little evidence that if the same two samples were rearrayed the results would be similar.

Even more important, the conclusions derived from comparing two RNA samples, even if they are arrayed on replicate arrays, apply only to those two samples and not to the tissues or experimental conditions from which they were derived. For example, in comparing two RNA samples, none of the biological variability is represented. In comparing expression profiles of tumors of one type to tumors of another type, there is generally substantial variation among tumors of the same class (e.g., Hedenfalk et al. 2001). There may even be substantial variation in expression within a single tumor. Hence, comparison of one RNA sample from one tumor of the first type to one RNA sample from one tumor of the second type is not adequate. In comparing tissue from inbred strains of mice, the biological variability is generally less than for human tissue but some biological replication is still necessary. Even for comparing expression of a cell line under two conditions, there is biological variability resulting from variation in experimental conditions, growth and harvest of the cells, and extraction of the RNA. Hence some replication of the entire experiment is important. This is discussed further in the next section.

3.4 Sources of Variation and Levels of Replication

Some important sources of variation in microarray studies can be categorized as

- between individuals within the same "class" or between complete replication of tissue culture experiments under the same experimental conditions;
- between specimens from the same individual or same experiment;
- between RNA samples from the same specimen;
- between arrays for the same RNA sample;
- between replicate spots on the same array.

Replicate arrays made from the same sample of RNA are often called *technical replicates*, in contrast to *biological replicates* made from RNA from biologically independent samples (Yang and Speed 2002b). There are, however, several levels of biological replicates.

Suppose we wish to determine gene expression differences between breast tumors with a mutated BRCA1 gene and tumors without a mutation. If we performed array experiments on one breast tumor with a BRCA1 mutation and one without a mutation we would not be able to draw any valid conclusions about the relationship of BRCA1 mutations to gene expression because we have no information about the natural variation within the two populations being studied. The situation would not improve even if the tumors under investigation were large enough for us to be able to perform multiple mRNA extractions and run independent array hybridizations on each extraction. Sets of tumors representative of the BRCA1 mutated population and the non-BRCA1 mutated population are necessary to draw valid conclusions about the relationship of BRCA1 mutations to gene expression.

There is sometimes confusion with regard to the level of replication appropriate for microarray studies. For example, in comparing expression profiles of BRCA1 mutated tumors to expression profiles of non-BRCA1mutated tumors, it is not necessary to have replicate arrays of a single RNA sample extracted from a single biopsy of a single tumor. Having such replication may provide protection from having to exclude the tumor if the one array available is of poor quality, but such replications are merely assay replicates and do not satisfy the crucial need for studying multiple tumors of each type. Often the biological variation between individuals will be much larger than the assay variation and it will be inefficient to perform replicate arrays using specimens from a small number of individuals rather than performing single arrays using a larger number of individuals.

In comparing expression profiles between two cell lines, or for a given cell line under different conditions, the concept of "individual" may be unclear. Suppose, for example, we wish to compare the expression profile of a cell line before treatment to the expression profile after treatment. Cell lines change their expression profiles depending on the culture conditions. Growing the cells and harvesting the RNA under "fixed conditions" will result in variable expression profiles because of differences in important factors such as the confluence state of the culture at the time of cell harvesting. Consequently, it is important to have independent biological replicates of the complete experiment under each of the conditions being compared. The degree of variation between independent biological samples may be less for experiments involving cell lines or inbred strains of model species compared to those involving human tissue samples, and this will influence the number of biological samples required as described in Section 3.8.

In some cases it is useful to obtain two specimens from the same individual. For example, if you are attempting to discover a new taxonomy of a disease based on an expression profile, it is useful to establish that the classification is robust to sampling variation within the same individual. For many studies of human tissue, however, the tissue samples will not be large enough to provide multiple specimens for independent processing. It is important to note that there is a distinction between multiple specimens from the same individual and multiple independently labeled aliquots of one RNA sample. The latter will show less variability than the former, especially when the tissue is heterogeneous. However, even without tissue heterogeneity, variation may be observed among expression profiles of multiple specimens taken from the same individual because of differences in tissue handling and RNA extraction.

Performing technical replicate arrays with independently labeled aliquots of the same RNA provides information about the reproducibility of the microarray assay, that is, the reproducibility of the labeling, hybridization, and quantification procedures. It is useful to know that the reagents, protocols and procedures used provide reproducible results on aliquots of the same RNA sample. Generally, it will be sufficient to obtain such technical replicates on just a few RNA samples. Serious attention should be devoted to reduce technical variability in a study. If possible, RNA extraction, labeling, and hybridization of all arrays in an experiment should be performed by the same individual using the same reagents. If spotted arrays are used, it is desirable to use arrays from the same print set and certainly the same batch of internal reference RNA. If samples become available at different times in a long-term study, it is best to save frozen specimens so that all of the array assays can be done at approximately the same time.

When technical replicate arrays of the same RNA samples are obtained, they can be averaged to improve precision of the estimate of the expression profile for a given RNA sample. If reproducibility is poor, however, it may be preferable to discard technically inferior arrays rather than average replicates. Although averaging of replicates may seem ad hoc, analysis of variance methods also average replicates although they account for the differences in precision available for different samples based on their possibly varying number of replicates. Replicate arrays of the same RNA samples are also sometimes used in dye-swap experimental designs described later in this chapter.

3.5 Pooling of Samples

Some investigators pool samples in the hope that through pooling they can reduce the number of microarrays needed. For example, in comparing two tissue types, a pool of one type of tissue is compared to a pool of the other tissue type. Replicate arrays might be performed on each pooled sample. Although the pooled sample approach may be applicable for preliminary screening, the approach does not provide a valid basis for biological conclusions about the types of tissues being compared. If only one array of each pooled sample is prepared, then even the two pools cannot be validly statistically compared because there is no estimate of the variability associated with independently labeling and hybridizing the same pool onto different arrays. Even if the two pools are hybridized to replicate arrays, one cannot assess the variability among pools of the same type and so one doesn't know how adequate a pool of that number of RNA specimens is in reflecting the population of that tissue type. Unless multiple biologically independent pools (of distinct specimens) of each type are arrayed, only the pooled samples themselves can be compared, not the populations from which they were derived. Biological replication is necessary. It can be achieved either by assaying individual samples, or by assaying independent pools of distinct samples. Studying independent pools of samples would be necessary in studying small model species where it may be necessary to pool in order to obtain enough RNA for assay (Jin et al. 2001).

3.6 Pairing Samples on Dual-Label Microarrays

With Affymetrix GeneChips^{TM}, single samples are labeled and hybridized to individual arrays. Spotted cDNA arrays, however, generally use a dual-label system in which two RNA samples are separately labeled, mixed, and hybridized together to each array. When using dual-label arrays one must decide on a design for pairing and labeling samples.

3.6.1 The Reference Design

The most commonly used design, called the reference design, uses an aliquot of a reference RNA as one of the samples hybridized to each array. This serves as an internal standard so that the intensity of hybridization to a probe for a sample of interest is measured relative to the intensity of hybridization to the same probe on the same array for the reference sample. This relative hybridization intensity produces a value that is standardized against variation in size and shape of corresponding spots on different arrays. Relative intensity is also automatically standardized with regard to variation in sample distribution across each array inasmuch as the two samples are mixed and therefore distributed similarly. The measure of relative hybridization generally used is the logarithm of the ratio of intensities of the two labeled specimens at the probe. Figure 3.1 is taken from Brody et al. (2002) who cohybridized labeled RNA from C2C12 myoblast cells and from 10T1/2 fibroblasts on an array that contained 100 spots for the glycerol-3-phosphate dehydrogenase gene. The figure shows the vast range of intensities among spots printed with the same clone on the same array. The ratio of intensities for the two samples, however, has little variation as evidenced by the tight linear association.

The reference design is illustrated in Figure 3.2. Generally, the reference is labeled with the same dye on each array. Any gene specific dye bias not removed by normalization affects all arrays similarly and does not bias class comparisons. Using a reference design, any subset of samples can be compared to any other subset of samples. Hence the design is not dependent on the specification of a single type of class comparison. For example, in studying BRCA1 mutated and BRCA1 nonmutated tumors, one might be interested in comparing samples based on their mutation status, comparing samples based

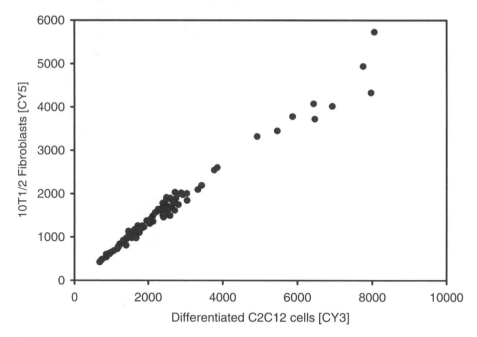

Fig. 3.1. Intensities of labeled RNA from C2C12 myoblast cells and labeled RNA from 10T1/2 fibroblasts hybridized to one array containing 100 spots of the glycerol-3-phosphate dehydrogenase gene. The figure shows the vast range of intensities among spots printed with the same clone on the same array. The ratio of intensities for the two samples, however, has little variation. From Brody et al. (2002).

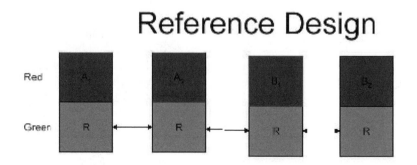

Fig. 3.2. Reference design. Aliquot of reference sample is labeled with the same label and used on each array.

on their estrogen receptor status, or comparing samples based on the stage of disease of the patient. The reference design is also convenient for class discovery using cluster analysis because the relative expression measurements are consistently measured with respect to the same reference sample.

If a laboratory uses reference designs with the same reference sample for all of their arrays, even those for different experiments, then all of their expression profiles can be directly compared. Consequently, expression signatures of different tissues studied in different experiments can be compared. This latter advantage can even extend to comparisons of expression profiles made by different laboratories using reference designs with the same reference sample.

There is sometimes confusion about the role of the reference sample. Some investigators erroneously believe that analysis is always based on combining single array determinations of whether the Cy5 (red) label is differentially expressed compared to the Cy3 (green) label for a given spot on a given array. Therefore they assume that the reference sample must be biologically relevant for comparison to the nonreference samples. In fact, the reference sample does not need to have any biological relevance. The analysis will usually involve quantitative comparisons of the average logarithm of intensity ratios for one set of arrays to average log ratios for another set of arrays.

It is desirable that most of the genes be expressed in the reference sample but not expressed at so high a level as to saturate the intensity detection system. Often, the reference sample consists of a mixture of cell lines so that nearly all genes will be expressed to some level. It is also important that a single batch of reference RNA is used for all arrays in a reference design. Different batches of reference RNA may have quite different expression profiles. When assaying samples collected over a long period of time, it is generally best to freeze the RNA samples and to perform the microarray assays at one time when all reagents can be standardized.

3.6.2 The Balanced Block Design

A disadvantage of the reference design is that half of the hybridizations are used for the reference sample, which may be of no real interest. Balanced block designs (Dobbin and Simon 2002) are alternatives that can be used in simple situations. For example, suppose one wished to compare BRCA1 mutated breast tumors to BRCA1 nonmutated breast tumors, that equal numbers of each tumor were available and that no other comparisons or other analyses were of interest. One could hybridize on each array one BRCA1 mutated tumor sample with one nonmutated sample. On half of the arrays the BRCA1 mutated tumors should be labeled with the red dye and on the other half the nonmutated tumors should be labeled with the red dye. This block design is illustrated in Figure 3.3. The analysis of data for the block design is discussed in Section 7.9. In its simplest form, a paired value t-test or Wilcoxon signed-rank test is performed for each gene, pairing the samples cohybridized to the same array. The block design can accommodate n samples of each type using

Balanced Block Design

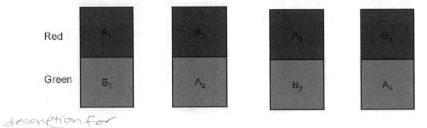

descnption for

Fig. 3.3. Loop design for comparing two classes of samples. Each biologically independent sample is subaliquoted and hybridized to two arrays, once with the Cy3 label and once with the Cy5 label. Each array contains a sample from each class.

only n microarrays. No reference RNA is used at all. The reference design would require $2n$ arrays to accommodate n nonreference samples from each of the two classes.

The balanced block design is very efficient in the use of arrays, but it has major limitations. For one, cluster analysis of the expression profiles cannot be performed effectively. Without a common reference, any comparisons between expression profiles of samples on different arrays will be subject to noise resulting from variation in size and shape of corresponding spots on different arrays and variation in sample distribution patterns on individual arrays (Dobbin and Simon 2002).

Another important limitation of the balanced block design is that it is based on a single specified two-class comparison. It does not easily accommodate analyzing the data in different ways for contrasting different groups of samples. Because it may be difficult to pair the samples simultaneously with regard to all of the class comparisons of interest, the block design is most effective when there is a single type of class comparison. The block design is also not effective for developing class predictors as described in Chapter 8.

In addition, the balanced block design also requires an arbitrary pairing of samples from the two classes and is less effective than the reference design when there is large intersample variability or when the number of samples, rather than the number of arrays, is limiting (Dobbin and Simon 2002).

3.6.3 The Loop Design

Loop designs (Kerr and Churchill 2001a) are another alternative to reference designs. When cluster analysis is planned, two aliquots of each sample must be arrayed for the loop design (Figure 3.4). For example, the first array would consist of one aliquot of the first sample labeled red and an aliquot of the second sample labeled green. The second array would consist of a second aliquot of the second sample, labeled red this time, and an aliquot of a third sample

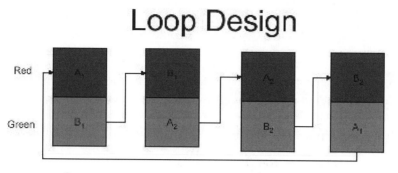

description for

← **Fig. 3.4.** Balanced block design for comparing two classes of samples. Each array contains a biologically independent sample from each class. Each class is labeled on half the arrays with one label and on the other half of the arrays with the other label. Each biologically independent sample is hybridized to a single array.

labeled green. The third array would consist of a second aliquot of the third sample labeled red this time, and an aliquot of a fourth sample labeled green. This loop continues and concludes with the nth and final array which consists of a second aliquot of the final sample n labeled red and hybridized with a second aliquot of the first sample, labeled green this time. This uses n arrays to study n samples, using two aliquots of each sample. The loops permit all pairs of samples to be contrasted in a manner that controls for variation in spot size and sample distribution patterns using a statistical model. Contrasting two samples far apart in the loop, however, involves modeling many indirect effects corresponding to the arrays linking the two arrays of interest and this adds substantial variance to many of these contrasts (Dobbin and Simon 2002). Consequently loop designs are not effective for cluster analysis. Loop designs can be used for class comparisons, but are less efficient than balanced block designs and require more complex methods of analysis than do common reference designs. Loop designs are less robust against the presence of bad quality arrays; two bad arrays break the loop. Loop designs also require enough RNA to be available for each sample for at least two hybridizations. Because of these limitations, loop designs are not generally recommended.

3.7 Reverse Labeling (Dye Swap)

Some investigators believe that all arrays should be performed both forward- and reverse- labeled. That is, for an array with sample A labeled with Cy3 and sample B labeled with Cy5, there should be another array with sample A labeled with Cy5 and sample B labeled with Cy3. In general, this is unnecessary and wasteful of resources (Dobbin et al. 2003a,b). Balanced labeling, as described in Section 3.6.2 is in general much more efficient than replicating hybridizations of the same specimens with swapped dye labeling. We discuss here, however, one circumstance where some reverse-labeling of samples is appropriate.

Dye swap or dye balance issues arise because the relative labeling intensity of the Cy3 and Cy5 may be different for different genes. Although the normalization process may remove average dye bias, gene-specific dye bias may remain. This is not important for comparing classes of nonreference samples using a reference design when the reference is consistently assigned the same label. Suppose, however, that we wanted to compare tumor tissue to matched normal tissue from the same patient using dual-label microarrays. As discussed in Section 3.6.2, one effective design would be to pair tumor and normal tissues from the same patient for cohybridization on the same array, with half of these arrays having the tumor labeled with Cy3 and the other half having the tumor labeled with Cy5 (Figure 3.3). Because the dye assignments are balanced, it is not necessary to perform any reverse-labeled replicate arrays of the tissues from the same patient (Dobbin et al. 2003a,b). For a fixed total number of arrays, it is best to use the available arrays to assay tissue from new patients, using the balanced block design described, rather than to perform replicate reverse-labeled arrays for single patients. The balanced block design is also best when there are n tumor tissues and n normal tissues even though the tissues are not from the same patients, or for comparing any two classes of samples. In these cases, the samples may be randomly paired, or paired based on balance with regard to potentially confounding variables such as the age of the specimens.

In some cases a reference design is used in which the primary objective is comparison of classes of the nonreference samples but comparison to the internal reference is a secondary objective. For example, there may be several types of transgenic mouse breast tumors for comparison and the internal reference may be a pool of normal mouse breast epithelium. Because the primary interest is comparison among multiple tumors models, a reference design may be chosen. The use of a pool of normal breast epithelium as the internal reference, rather than a mixture of cell lines, reflects some interest in comparison of expression profiles in tumors relative to normal breast epithelium. Comparison to a pool of normal breast epithelium is somewhat problematic, however, for reasons described previously in Section 3.5. The conclusions derived from comparison of the tumor samples to the internal reference will apply to that pool of normal epithelium, but it will not be possible to evaluate how representative that pool is. Nevertheless, the comparison may be of interest.

In order to ensure that the comparison of tumor expression to that of the reference is not distorted by gene-specific dye bias when using a reference design, some reverse-labeled arrays are needed. One can then fit a statistical analysis of variance model to the logarithms of the intensities for each channel as described in Section 7.9. Not all arrays need to be reverse-labeled; 5 to10 reverse-labeled pairs of arrays will generally be adequate. Except for this purpose of comparison of experimental samples to the common reference in a reference design, however, Dobbin et al. (2003a,b) recommend against reverse-labeling of the same two RNA samples.

3.8 Number of Biological Replicates Needed

As indicated in Section 3.3, it is not generally meaningful to compare expression profiles in two RNA samples without biological replication. The number of independent biological samples needed depends on the objectives of the experiment. We describe here a relatively straightforward method for planning sample size for testing whether a particular gene is differentially expressed between two predefined classes. Such a test can be applied to each gene if we adjust for the number of comparisons involved (Simon et al. 2002).

This approach to sample size planning may be used for dual-label arrays using reference designs or for single-label oligonucleotide arrays. For dual-label arrays the expression level for a gene is the log ratio of intensity relative to the reference sample; for Affymetrix GeneChip^{TM} arrays it is usually the log signal, discussed in Chapter 4. The approach to sample size planning described here is based on the assumption that the expression measurements are approximately normally distributed among samples of the same class. Let σ denote the standard deviation of the expression level for a gene among samples within the same class and suppose that the means of the two classes differ by δ for that gene. For example, with base 2 logarithms, a value of $\delta = 1$ corresponds to a twofold difference between classes. We assume that the two classes will be compared with regard to the level of expression of each gene and that a statistically significant difference will be declared if the null hypothesis can be rejected at a significance level α. The *significance level* is the probability of concluding that the gene is differentially expressed between the two classes when in fact the means are the same ($\delta = 0$). The significance level α will be set stringently in order to limit the number of false positive findings inasmuch as thousands of genes will be analyzed. The desired statistical power will be denoted $1 - \beta$. *Statistical power* is the probability of obtaining statistical significance in comparing gene expression between the two classes when the true difference in mean expression levels between the classes is δ. Statistical power is one minus the false negativity rate (β).

Under these conditions, the total number of samples required from different individuals or different replications of the experiment approximately satisfies the equation:

$$n = \frac{4\left(t_{\alpha/2} + t_\beta\right)^2}{(\delta/\sigma)^2}, \tag{3.1}$$

where $t_{\alpha/2}$ and t_β denote the $(100)\alpha/2$ and 100β percentiles of the t distribution with $n - 2$ degrees of freedom. Because the t percentiles depend on n, however, the equation can only be solved iteratively. When the number of samples n is sufficiently large, Equation (3.1) can be adequately approximated by

$$n = \frac{4\left(z_{\alpha/2} + z_\beta\right)^2}{(\delta/\sigma)^2}, \tag{3.2}$$

where $z_{\alpha/2}$ and z_β denote the corresponding percentiles of the standard normal distribution (Desu et al. 1990). The normal percentiles do not depend on n, and hence equation (3.2) can be solved directly for n. For example, for $\alpha = 0.001$ and $\beta = 0.05$ as recommended below, the standard normal percentiles are $z_{\alpha/2} = -3.29$ and $z_\beta = -1.645$, respectively. Expressions (3.1) and (3.2) give the total number of biologically independent samples needed for comparing the two classes; $n/2$ should be selected from each class.

The fact that expression levels for many genes will be examined indicates that the size of α should be much smaller than 0.05. The 0.05 value is only appropriate for experiments where the focus is on a single endpoint or single test. If $\alpha = 0.05$ is used for testing the differential expression of 10,000 genes between two classes, then even if none of the genes is truly differentially expressed, one would expect 500 false discoveries; that is, 500 false claims of statistical significance. The expected number of false discoveries is α times the number of genes that are nondifferentially expressed. This is true regardless of the correlation pattern among the genes.

In order to keep the number of false discoveries manageable with thousands of genes analyzed, $\alpha = 0.001$ is often appropriate. For example, using $\alpha = 0.001$ with 10,000 genes gives 10 expected false discoveries. This is much less conservative than the multi-test adjustment procedures used for clinical trials where the probability of even one false discovery is limited to 5%. We recommend $\beta = 0.05$ in order to have good statistical power for identifying genes that really are differentially expressed. If the ratio of sample sizes in the two groups is $k{:}1$ instead of $1{:}1$, then the total sample size increases by a factor of $(k + 1)^2/4k$ compared to formula (3.2).

The parameter σ can usually be estimated based on data showing the degree of variation of expression values among similar biological tissue samples. σ will vary among genes. For log ratio expression levels, we have seen the median values of σ of approximately 0.5 (using base 2 logarithms) for human tissue samples and similar values for Affymetrix GeneChips^{TM}. The parameter δ represents the size of the difference between the two classes we wish to be able to detect. For $\log_2$ ratios or $\log_2$ signals, $\delta = 1$ is corresponds to a twofold difference in expression level between classes. This value of δ is reasonable because differences of less than twofold are difficult to measure reproducibility with microarrays. Using $\alpha = 0.001$, $\beta = 0.05$, $\delta = 1$ and $\sigma = 0.50$ in (3.2) gives a required sample size of approximately 26 total samples, or 13 in each of the two classes. The more accurate formula (3.1) gives a requirement of 30 total samples, or 15 in each of the two classes.

The within-class variability depends somewhat on the type of specimens; human tissue samples have greater variability than inbred strains of mice or than cell lines. In experiments studying microarrays of kidney tissue for inbred strains of mice, the median standard deviation of log ratios for a normal kidney was approximately 0.25, with little variation among genes. For cell line data on Affymetrix GeneChips^{TM}, we have seen similar standard deviations for $\log_2$ signals. Using $\alpha = 0.001$, $\beta = 0.05$, $\delta = 1$ and $\sigma = 0.25$ in formula (3.1) gives a required sample size of 11 total samples. Because we cannot have 5.5 samples per class, we should round up to 6 samples per class. If this were a time-series experiment with more than two time points, then one should plan for 6 animals per timepoint in order to enable expression profiles to be compared for all pairs of time points.

The discussion above applies either to dual-label arrays using a reference design and log ratio as the measure of relative expression, or to single-label arrays such as the Affymetrix GeneChip^{TM} arrays using log transformed signals or another measure of expression. When dual-label arrays are used with the block design to compare either naturally paired or independent samples from two classes, then the same formulas apply but the definition of σ changes. For the block design, σ represents the standard deviation of variation across arrays of the log ratio computed with one sample from each class (Dobbin et al. 2003). Preliminary data are generally needed to estimate σ.

Many of the considerations for comparing predefined classes also apply to identifying genes that are significantly associated with patient outcome (Simon et al. 2002). When the outcome is survival and not all patients are followed until death, the analogue of expression (3.2) is

$$E = \frac{(z_{\alpha/2} + z_\beta)^2}{(\tau \ln(\delta))^2}. \tag{3.3}$$

E denotes the number of events (e.g., deaths) that need to be observed in order to achieve the targeted statistical power. For survival comparisons, the statistical power often depends on the number of events, rather than the number of patients. For a given number of patients accrued, the number of events will increase as the duration of followup increases. There is a tradeoff between number of patients accrued and duration of followup in order to achieve a targeted number of events. In expression (3.3), τ denotes the standard deviation of the log ratio or log signal for the gene over the entire set of samples. δ represents the hazard ratio associated with a one-unit change in the log ratio or log signal and ln denotes the natural logarithm. Note that we are assuming that the log ratio or log signal values are based on logarithms to the base 2, so a one-unit change in the expression level represents a twofold change.

If $\tau = 0.5$ and $\delta = 2$, then 203 events are required for a two-sided significance level of 0.001 and power of 0.95. This makes for a large study in most cases because to observe 203 events in a group of patients with a 50% event rate requires 406 patients. The large number of events results from assuming that a doubling of hazard rate requires a two standard deviation change in log ratio. Hence most patients would have expression levels that had very limited effects on survival. Therefore it may be more reasonable to size the study for detecting statistically significant differences in only the more variable genes, for example, $\tau = 1$ and $\delta = 2$, which results in 51 required events. Genes that have small standard deviations across the entire set of samples are difficult to use for prognostic prediction in clinical situations.

The multivariate permutation tests described in Chapter 7 are a more powerful method for finding differentially expressed genes than the univariate parametric test that is the basis for formulas (3.1) and (3.2). Nevertheless, the sample size formulas given here are useful for planning purposes and provide control of the number of false discoveries in a reasonable manner. Other methods have been described by Black and Doerge (2002), Lee and Whitmore, (2002), and Pan et al. (2002). Adequate methods for determining the number of samples required for gene expression studies whose objectives are class prediction or class discovery have not yet been developed. Hwang et al. (2002) provide a method of planning sample size to test the hypothesis that the classes are completely equivalent with regard to expression profile. The sample size formulas given above provide reasonable minimum sample sizes for class prediction studies. Often, however, developing multivariate class predictors or survival predictors involves extensive analyses beyond determining the genes that are informative univariately. Consequently, larger sample sizes are generally needed for class prediction studies (Rosenwald et al. 2002).

In class prediction studies it is important to estimate the misclassification rate of the identified multivariate predictor. There is a problem using the same data to develop a prediction model and to estimate the accuracy of the model, particularly when the number of candidate predictors is orders of magnitude larger than the number of cases (Simon et al. 2003). Consequently, special methods of analysis must be used to provide unbiased estimates of prediction accuracy. One approach is to split the data into a training set and a validation set (Rosenwald et al. 2002). Other approaches involve more sophisticated methods such as cross-validation or bootstrap resampling (discussed in Chapter 8). Cross-validation and bootstrap resampling can be used when the derivation of the prediction rule can be clearly defined as an algorithm with no subjective elements. In many cases, the derivation of the prediction rule is more complex and involves numerous analyses that cannot be easily specified in a manner that can automatically be applied to resampled datasets. In these cases, it is necessary to use the split sample approach to obtain an unbiased estimate of the accuracy of the class prediction rule. Initially the data are divided into a training set and a validation set. This division may be done randomly or may be balanced by factors such as an institution contributing the specimens. The validation set is put aside and not analyzed at all until a completely specified prediction rule is defined based on analyses conducted using the training set. The prediction rule resulting from the analysis should be completely specified, including the estimation of parameters and the establishment of threshold values for class prediction. After the analysis of the training set is completed, the validation set is unlocked and the completely specified prediction rule is applied to the cases in the validation set. The prediction accuracy is determined based on the performance of the predictor on the validation set. Usually about one third to one half of the total dataset is reserved for the validation set. Therefore in planning the size of a class prediction study that will use the split sample approach, it should be recognized that perhaps only half of the data will be available for development of the multivariate predictor.

Often investigators use validation sets that are far too small to provide meaningful validation. Table 3.1 shows the upper 95% confidence limit for the misclassification rate as a function of the observed proportion of misclassified specimens and the number of specimens in the validation set. Suppose that the true misclassification rate is 10% and you are lucky enough to observe no misclassifications in the validation set. With only 10 specimens in the validation set you would be able to bound the true misclassification rate to be no greater than 26%. But it is just as likely that you would obtain 20% of the validation set misclassified. In this case, even with 50 samples in the validation set, you would only be able to bound the true misclassification rate to be no greater than 32%. Consequently, a substantial validation set is needed in order to adequately estimate the true misclassification rate.

Table 3.1.

Number of Validation Samples	Upper 95% Confidence Limit for Misclassification Rate	
	None Misclassified in Validation Set (%)	20% Misclassified in Validation Set (%)
5	45	66
10	26	51
20	14	40
50	6	32

4

Image Analysis

After hybridization of fluorescently labeled cDNA molecules to the microarray, the array is stimulated with a laser and the intensity of fluorescence is measured at a dense grid of pixel locations on the array. An image file is created that stores all of the pixel-level intensities. There are many more pixels than probes on the array. Image analysis is the procedure by which pixel level data are processed and converted to measures of intensity for the arrayed probes. There are several image analysis methods available and it is useful for the investigator to have some understanding of the approaches used.

We begin with a brief description of how images of gene expression arrays are created. Then we describe the main steps of image analysis: gridding, segmentation, background correction, feature (signal) intensity extraction, and flagging spots for exclusion. Because the methods used for cDNA microarrays and Affymetrix GeneChip^{TM} arrays are different, we discuss the above steps for the two types of arrays separately.

4.1 Image Generation

A scanner (laser scanning confocal microscope) or a charge-coupled device (CCD) camera is used to quantify the intensity of fluorescence at each pixel location on the microarray. These intensities are saved in a file formatted as a 16 bit tagged image file (TIFF). The fluorescent dye molecules hybridized to the probes emit photons when stimulated by a laser. Emission wavelengths differ for the two dyes, thus the emitted photons can be selectively filtered to allow quantification of the amount emitted by each dye. For cDNA microarrays, the dyes Cy3 and Cy5 have emission wavelengths in the 510 to 550 nm and 630 to 660 nm ranges, respectively. With commonly used scanners, the emitted light is captured by a photomultiplier tube (PMT) detector in the scanner and converted into electric current. The PMT's voltage can be adjusted in each channel to maximize the dynamic range of the scanner with minimal saturation of pixels and also to get balanced intensities between the two channels. Pixels are saturated when more photons are detected than the PMT can process or when the output of the PMT exceeds the range of the analogue-to-digital converter. Saturated pixels are displayed as white pixels in the image. The differences in amplification resulting from PMT voltage adjustment will lead to changes in signal intensity, but this should not affect results for the majority of genes (except for the saturated spots) after proper normalization (see Chapter 6). The intensity for each probe is proportional to the number of molecules of the fluorescent label in DNA bound to the probe.

4.2 Image Analysis for cDNA Microarrays

4.2.1 Image Display

Figure 2.2 shows a typical cDNA microarray image. It has two rows and two columns of blocks called subgrids, which are uniformly spaced. Each subgrid consists of several rows and columns of spots. An enlarged image of one spot patch is shown in Figure 4.1, and the smallest discernable element in that enlarged image is called a pixel. The raw intensities for each of the two channels are saved as 16 bit binary integers. They can be displayed as images with pixel values ranging from 0 to 65,535 shades of grey. The darkest black pixels represent low-intensity value and the bright white pixels represent high-intensity value. For purposes of visual display, the two separate 16 bit TIFF files are frequently combined and saved as a 24 bit composite RGB (red-green-blue) image. In this RGB composite, each of the three color channels is composed of only an 8 bit image. In order to be displayed as a 24 bit composite RGB overlay image, the raw images must first be reduced from 16 bits to 8 bits using an image compression method. Then the image from Cy3 is placed in the green channel, the image from Cy5 is placed in the red channel, and the blue channel is set to 0. For image analysis the original 16 bit TIFF files are used.

4.2.2 Gridding

The first step in array image analysis is to overlay a rectangular grid onto the pixels in a manner that isolates each spot within a cell. *Gridding* is usually a semi or fully automated process that takes advantage of the fact that robotic spotting is performed in a regular predetermined manner. Most software systems begin by estimating the overall position of the array in the image, the separation between rows and columns of grids, the spacing of spots within each grid, and translation of individual grids or spots. For example, GenePix (Axon 2001) automatically generates grids using the printing information (grid configuration), and then provides a manual fine-tuning option.

4.2.3 Segmentation

Gridding establishes the location of a rectangular *patch* that contains the spot. The second step, *segmentation*, involves identifying the pixels within the patch that are contained in the spot. This set of pixels is called the *foreground region* or *spot mask*. Several different segmentation algorithms are in common use for this purpose.

Fixed or adaptive circle segmentation is based on approximating the foreground region by a circle. Fixed circle segmentation uses the same circle diameter for all spots. Adaptive circle segmentation uses the intensity data to estimate the best diameter separately for each spot. However, both approaches are of limited accuracy inasmuch as real spots have irregular shapes (Figure 4.1) because of printing, hybridization, and slide surface chemistry factors.

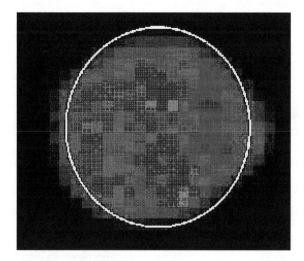

Fig. 4.1. An enlarged spot patch shown at pixel level. The spot is noncircular shaped, with a circular mask placed for segmentation.

To address the problems caused by spot irregularities, adaptive segmentation methods such as watershed and seeded region growing have been applied (Beucher and Meyer 1993; Adams and Bischof 1994). The watershed algorithm is applied separately to each spot patch. The pixels in a spot patch are partitioned into disjoint watershed sets. All the pixels in the same watershed set "drain" into the same local minimum with regard to the distribution of pixel intensities. The definition of watersheds is as follows. For each point in the spot patch, a path is determined by choosing the direction of the steepest descent with respect to intensity. These paths lead to local minima. All pixels that have a path leading to the same minimum belong to the same catchment basin and together constitute one segment. The borders between touching segments are the watersheds. The average intensity in each segment is computed, and the segments with largest average intensities are taken as the foreground region. This region need not be contiguous or regular.

The seeded region growing (SRG) algorithm is another method for representing irregular foreground regions. SRG is based on choosing a small number of high-intensity pixels as the initial seeds. The region defined by each seed is enlarged contiguously to contain other relatively high-intensity pixels. When a region cannot be further enlarged without introducing pixels with intensity below some specified threshold criterion, growth of that segment ceases. The resulting segments of high-intensity pixels are taken as the foreground region.

Histogram segmentation is another commonly used method. It does not rely on spatial information. Instead, the histogram of intensities for pixels within each spot patch is computed. Threshold percentiles are then used to define the foreground and background regions; for example, pixels in the 5th to 20th percentiles of the intensity distribution are often chosen for the background, and pixels in the 80th to 95th percentiles are chosen for the foreground. A non-spatial segmentation method based on the Mann-Whitney test has also been proposed (Chen et al. 1997).

4.2.4 Foreground Intensity Extraction

Once the foreground and background regions are determined for each spot, the pixel values are summarized to give a single measurement for each region. Common summary values for the foreground include the mean or median value of the pixel intensities. The mean pixel intensity has the appeal of being directly related to the total (sum) of pixel intensities in the foreground. If spots are irregularly shaped and fixed or adaptive circle segmentation is used, the foreground region could include pixels not part of the probe leading to an underestimate of the true foreground intensity. However, this downward bias is corrected when the ratio of the two channel background-adjusted intensities is calculated.

Occasionally, spots contain a few aberrantly high pixel intensities due to artifacts and these may tend to distort the mean value. For this reason, some investigators prefer to summarize the foreground pixels by the median pixel intensity. Although more robust to aberrant pixels, the median has the disadvantage of not being directly related to the total intensity. Also, if spots are very elongated ovals or have large "holes" covering more than 50% of the pixels in the circular mask applied in fixed or adaptive circle segmentation, the median value may be equal to background intensity, totally missing the signal. The trimmed mean may be a better alternative than the median. A $k\%$ trimmed mean is the mean calculated after excluding the largest (or smallest) k percentage of the pixel intensity values.

Methods that allow flexibility in spot shape such as histogram or adaptive methods have the potential of better estimating total intensity of bound label. Nevertheless, calculating the mean foreground with fixed or adaptive circles is relatively simple and seems to work well in practice. Comparisons performed by Yang et al. (2002c) indicated that the differences among the algorithms had very small impact on foreground intensity values.

4.2.5 Background Correction

Considering nonspecific binding and auto-fluorescence, it seems clear that the foreground intensity would be more properly proportional to abundance of bound labeled cDNA if an accurate adjustment for background fluorescence could be performed. Currently, there are different approaches to background adjustment, and studies have shown that the choice of background adjustment method can have a large impact on the final output such as log ratios (Yang et al. 2002c; Jain et al. 2002).

Global background correction uses the same constant to represent the background for all spots. This constant can be calculated by using a set of negative control spots. Alternatively, one can use a low percentile (e.g. third percentile) of all the pixel intensities as the background level. Brown et al. (2001) computed a global background estimate as part of their normalization procedure to make the average ratio across the array as close to one as possible. However, global estimation does not take into account the local background variations that exist in many cases.

Regional background correction provides greater flexibility than global correction (Axon 2001; Yang et al. 2001; Jain et al. 2002). For example, the algorithm used by GenePix is based on a circle centered on each spot. The region from which the background is calculated for any spot has a diameter that is three times the diameter of the circle used to define the foreground for that spot. Pixels contained within the large circle that are not within any foreground region and are not wholly inside a two-pixel wide ring around the foreground circle of the current spot are used to compute the background for the current spot.

Yang et al. (2001) applied an algorithm called morphological opening (Soille 1999) for background adjustment. Morphological opening is a method for obtaining a regionally smoothed estimate of the background for each spot without having to estimate the boundaries of the foreground regions of the spots. The algorithm is based on virtually moving a square structural element (SE) over the face of the array. The structural element is a window that is much larger than the size of any spot, but smaller than a grid of spots. When the SE is centered on a particular pixel, the intensity of that pixel is replaced by the minimum intensity of pixels covered by the SE. This is called the "erosion" step. After the erosion step is completed, the SE is again virtually moved over the face of the array in a "dilation" step. When the SE is centered on a pixel, the intensity of that pixel is replaced by the maximum of the values created during erosion for the pixels covered by the SE. The morphological opening filter removes all features that are not big enough to contain the structure element. By choosing a square structuring element much larger than the spot size, the operation removes all the spots and generates an image as an estimate of the background for the entire slide. Background for each spot is then calculated by sampling the estimated background image at the nominal centers of the spots. Compared with other background correction methods, morphological opening showed a low within- and between-slide variability in ratios in the study by Yang et al. (2002c), but there was no gold standard by which to evaluate whether the resulting estimates were more accurate.

Local background estimation may provide a poor estimate of nonspecific fluorescence because it may be highly variable if it is based on too small a region. Consequently, it is not uncommon for spots to have higher values for the background than for the foreground. Log ratios of background-adjusted signal values in the two channels are imprecise estimates of relative abundance of transcripts in the two samples for probes in which both of the background adjusted signals are extremely low. It may be better to exclude such probes from subsequent analysis. This is discussed further in Chapter 5.

4.2.6 Image Output File

For each spot and channel, the output file summarizes quantities such as foreground mean, median, and standard deviation of pixel intensities; background mean, median and standard deviation of pixel intensities; and the number of pixels in the foreground and background. The log base 2 ratio for each spot is:

$$\log_2 \frac{FR - BR}{FG - BG},\tag{4.1}$$

where FR and FG denote the foreground mean or median intensities of the red and green channels, and BR and BG denote the corresponding background mean or median intensities. Mean foreground intensities and median background intensities are recommended in most cases. The log ratio estimates the relative abundance of the corresponding gene transcripts in the two samples that were cohybridized to the array. Using the log ratio instead of the ratio makes the distribution more symmetrical and the variation less dependent on absolute signal magnitude. Most investigators use log ratios to do subsequent analysis. However, some methods such as ANOVA methods work on the log signal directly rather than on log ratios (Kerr and Churchill 2001a; Wolfinger et al. 2001; Dobbin et al. 2002, 2003).

Problematic spots should be flagged and omitted from the subsequent analysis. Image analysis packages provide the ability to flag individual spots automatically and manually, and flags are exported to the output file. Those spots include the ones not at the expected location, ones with a negative red or green signal after background subtraction, ones with too many saturated pixels, and ones with no hybridization.

4.3 Image Analysis for Affymetrix GeneChip™

GeneChip™ software analyzes the image data file (.dat) and computes a single intensity value for each probe cell on the array. The intensity data are saved to another file (.cel). Figure 4.2 represents a feature-level view of a high-density Affymetrix GeneChip™. Each gene has 16 to 20 probe pairs

Fig. 4.2. Feature view of Affymetrix GeneChip™.

that are scattered on the chip. Newer chips such as the Human Genome U133 Set, the Rat Expression Set 230, and Mouse Expression Set 430 have only 11 probe pairs per gene. For each probe pair, the upper perfect match (*PM*) probe usually gives a greater hybridization signal than its mismatch (*MM*) counterpart (Figure 4.3). However, it is possible that the *MM* probe sequence has high homology with another unknown sequence. Consequently, the mismatch probe may have even a greater signal than the perfect match probe. Control probes located at the corners of the probe array are used to align a grid to delineate the probe cells.

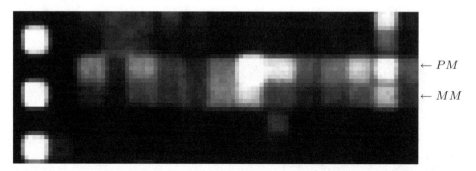

$\leftarrow PM$

$\leftarrow MM$

Fig. 4.3. Enlarged view of Affymetrix GeneChip^{TM}. Probe pairs appear as two bright stripes, with the upper stripe representing a perfect match (PM) probe and the corresponding mismatch (MM) probe directly beneath. Each grid represents a small region of the chip (typically 24 μm by 24 μm for the high density arrays and 50 μm by 50 μm for the low density arrays) containing 10^6 to 10^7 copies of a given probe.

GeneChip^{TM} software defines a feature intensity as the 75th percentile of the pixel intensities for that feature after removing the boundary pixels (Lockhart et al. 1996). Sometimes the bright intensities tend to blur the PM/MM boundary and result in an upward bias for the MM intensity. Schadt et al. (2001) proposed trimming pixel intensities more than three standard deviations from the mean pixel value within a feature.

Background correction is also necessary for the GeneChip^{TM} arrays. A high background implies that impurities, such as cell debris and salts, are binding to the array in a nonspecific manner and that these substances are fluorescing at 570 nm (the scanning wavelength). The GeneChip^{TM} software uses a regionalized method to do background subtraction. The array is first split into N rectangular zones (default 16). Within each zone, background intensities are calculated by averaging the lowest 2% of probe cell intensities, and background values are smoothed across the zones to obtain the cell-specific background estimates.

For the GeneChip^{TM} arrays, the average difference was the original way to produce gene-level summaries:

$$\frac{1}{n} \sum_i \left(PM_i - MM_i \right), \tag{4.2}$$

where n represents the total number of probe pairs for the gene, and PM_i and MM_i indicate the corresponding perfect match and mismatch probe intensities after background correction for the ith probe pair for the gene. In contrast to the relative quantification of hybridization represented by cDNA array-based ratios, the intensity values derived from GeneChip^{TM} arrays are considered to measure absolute hybridization. Any hybridization to the *MM* probe represents the level of nonspecific binding. Therefore it was thought that the intensity measured from the *MM* probe could be used as an estimate of cross-hybridization.

Since the above average difference measure frequently produced negative values, Affymetrix modified the algorithm in its Microarray Suite User Guide version 5. If the *MM* value is larger than the *PM* value for a probe pair, then the *MM* value is replaced by a smaller contrast value (*CT*). The *CT* value is based either on the average ratio between *PM* and *MM* for all of the probe pairs of that probe set, or (if that measure is too small) a value slightly smaller than *PM*. If the *MM* value is smaller than the corresponding *PM* value, then the *CT* value equals the *MM* value. The absolute expression value for probe set k is called the "signal log value" (SLV) and is defined as

$$SLV_k = Biweight\left\{\log_2(PM_{i,k} - CT_{i,k}) : i = 1, \ldots, n)\right\}, \qquad (4.3)$$

where *Biweight* stands for the one-step Tukey biweight function operating on the logs of the pairwise intensity differences between the *PM* and *MM* probe pairs for all of the n probe pairs in probe set k. The Tukey biweight algorithm (Hoaglin et al. 1983) is a method of robustly averaging values so as not to be heavily affected by outliers. It uses the median to define the center of the data. Then it uses the distance of each data point from the median to determine how much each value should contribute to the average. The signal value reported by the MAS software is a normalized signal and is described in Chapter 6.

Alternative methods for estimating the probe set summary signal are under active investigation (Efron et al. 2001; Li and Wong 2001a, b; Naef et al. 2001, Irizarry et al. 2003). Efron et al. (2001) proposed using partial *MM* values (half or one third) as rough estimates of cross-hybridization. A model-based approach for calculating gene summaries from probe level data was proposed by Li and Wong (2001a, b). For each gene k, they model the average differences in probe pair i for array j as $PM_{ij} - MM_{ij} = \theta_j\phi_i + \varepsilon_{ij}$. We have supressed use of the subscript k for ease of notation but separate models are fit for each gene k. The term θ_j represents an average expression index for the gene on array j, and the ϕ_i terms represent probe-specific sensitivities for probe pair i. The ε terms represent random experimental error. The probe-specific sensitivities are estimated using the data from all arrays in the experiment. These sensitivities indicate which probes of the probe set for gene k detect variations across the arrays and which do not. The array-specific expression index θ_j for a given gene k is estimated as a weighted linear combination of the $PM - MM$ differences for that probe set, with the probe sensitivity estimates being the weights. The Li and Wong method also provides confidence intervals for the expression index of each gene on each array and these intervals can be used for quality control purposes to distinguish the genes whose expression index is well determined from those in which it is not.

The issue of how to combine the *PM* and *MM* pairs to estimate an expression index for each gene on each array is still under intensive academic research. Some investigators even recommend using only the *PM* values and not the *MM* values in estimating the expression indices (Naef et al. 2001).

5

Quality Control

5.1 Introduction

Microarray signal intensities inherently contain a significant amount of noise. Usually the amount of noise in the signal is manageable and reliable conclusions can be made about the level of expression of a given probe. However, in certain cases there may be no reliable signal available or the noise dominates the signal. In these cases, it is advisable to either replace these values with an imputed value or else eliminate the probe from the analysis. In this chapter we discuss the circumstances under which an observation or set of observations should be excluded as well as methods of imputing values for excluded observations.

Determination of the acceptable amount of noise requires judgment on the part of the investigator. Many of the quality control suggestions in this chapter are of the form: Exclude a measured value should its quality fall below a certain threshold. We provide guidelines as to what reasonable thresholds might be, but these should not be considered the only acceptable thresholds. If the use of a particular set of thresholds leads to an unacceptable number of missing values, it might be reasonable to consider weakening the quality control standards. If, on the other hand, large numbers of outlier observations seem to be corrupting the analysis, it may be necessary to require greater stringency of quality control and raise the thresholds.

There are three levels at which quality control may be warranted: the probe level, the gene level and the array level. By poor probe quality, we mean poor quality of one particular gene expression measurement on one particular array. By poor gene quality, we mean poor quality of the expression measurement for a single gene across all arrays. By poor array quality, we mean poor quality of all spots on one particular glass slide or gene chip.

Sections 5.2 through 5.4 address quality control issues for two-color cDNA arrays. In section 5.5, we discuss which of these issues apply to the quality control of Affymetrix data.

5.2 Probe-Level Quality Control for Two-Color Arrays

In the case of two-color cDNA arrays, the probes will be the individual spots printed on the slide. Poor quality at the spot level on a given array can occur for a variety of reasons, some of which are technical such as a faulty printing, uneven distribution of the sample on the slide, or contamination with debris. Other reasons are related to the size of the signal relative to the noise. Because there are many ways in which a poorly measured spot can occur, there are multiple methods of detecting poorly measured spots. We recommend considering all of the following criteria, and eliminating or imputing any spot that fails any of them.

5.2.1 Visual Inspection of the Image File

Sometimes it is possible to notice anomalies on a slide by visually inspecting the array image file. Some arrays will have thin streaks of very high intensity that may cross through a number of spots (see Figure 5.1(a)). This may be caused by hairs or fibers being trapped on the slide, or scratches on the slide surface leading to a collection point for the sample that does not wash away. Any spot that comes in contact with such a streak will be of unusually high intensity, making its value highly suspect. All such spots should be flagged for exclusion or imputation.

A second common occurrence is the presence of air bubbles between the slide and cover slip. Because the sample never reaches these air pockets, they appear as dark regions on the image plot (see Figure 5.1(b)). Many of the spots inside the bubble will be excluded at the image analysis phase because no signal will be detected, but spots on the border of this region may be detected yet give a false reading. Therefore, we recommend that all spots that contact such a bubble be excluded

Another anomaly that may exist is a general green or red haze that covers an area of the slide (Figure 5.1(c),(d)). Many of these spots will likely be excluded for low signal-to-background ratio (discussed later in this section), and background subtraction may allow the remaining spots to be usable. As an added precaution, however, we recommend performing location-based normalization (Section 6.4) to adjust for any additional effect that may not be picked up by the background subtraction. If the haze is extremely bright and covers a large area of the slide (as in Figure 5.1(d)) it may be best to simply exclude the array. Along the top of Figure 5.1(c) there also appears to be an edge effect of bright red. Because this is very strong, but only affects a limited number of spots, we would exclude those spots along the top, keeping the rest of the array for analysis.

5.2.2 Spots Flagged at Image Analysis

Spot quality may deteriorate to the point that the image analysis software cannot identify the location of the particular spot and will flag the spot as

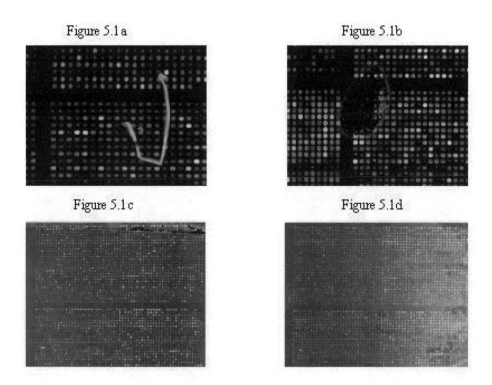

Figure 5.1a   Figure 5.1b

Figure 5.1c   Figure 5.1d

Fig. 5.1. Examples of array anomalies that can be detected through examination of the image file (a) Bright streak indicating the presence of a fiber on the array; (b) dark patch indicating the presence of a bubble on the array; (c) Background subtraction may be able to correct for the uniform green haze covering slide, but spots covered by red haze along top should be excluded; (d) Background subtraction alone may not be able to account for strong green haze on right side of slide. Location normalization is recommended.

not found. Because no spot is identified, it is clear that any values reported should not be used. Many image analysis software packages also provide their own systems for evaluating spot quality. These will often encompass some of the suggestions outlined below, so it is a good idea to eliminate spots that are flagged as poor quality by the software. Quality metrics that include several of the quality features discussed below are described by Wang et al. (2001) and Chen et al. (2002).

5.2.3 Spot Size

Most image analysis software report the number of foreground pixels used to determine the signal of a detected spot. Signals based on a very small number of pixels are likely to be poorly measured, and should be excluded. A reasonable threshold is to exclude spots whose foreground intensity in either channel was based on fewer than 25 pixels.

5.2.4 Weak Signal

In Chapter 4, we recommended converting the array signal intensities to log ratios prior to analysis. This conversion has an unfortunate side effect of increasing the effect of additive noise for small intensity values. As an example, consider that we have a gene that has equal expression in both channels; we would expect to find a log ratio equal to zero. Now suppose on one array we have good hybridization and find that the intensity in the channels is around 500, but that there was an additive error of ± 10. For example, suppose 510 was measured in the red channel and 490 was measured in the green channel so that we would obtain a log ratio of $\log_2(510/490) = 0.057$. In this case, we would correctly conclude that there was little difference between the channels. However, if the true signal in the red and green channel was around 20, then the same additive measurement error would lead to a log ratio of $\log_2(30/10) = 1.58$, indicating that the gene had a higher expression in the red channel than in the green channel. Furthermore, the error could be in the opposite direction, and we would incorrectly conclude the gene had higher expression in the green channel. For this reason, it is generally inadvisable to make any conclusions about spots that have low signals in both channels; such spots should be excluded. In practice, the vast majority of spots that are excluded from analysis are excluded for this reason.

If one channel has a strong signal and the other channel has a weak signal, then the situation is somewhat more complicated. Consider a spot that has a true intensity of 500 in the red channel and only 20 in the green channel. The true log ratio in this case will be $\log_2(500/20) = 4.64$. If there were an additive error of ± 10 then we would observe a log ratio between $\log_2(510/10) = 5.67$ and $\log_2(490/30) = 4.03$. Although there is a large amount of variability in the magnitude of such a signal, in both cases it is clear that there is much larger expression of the gene in the red channel than there is in the green channel and so there is useful information contained in the expression level of the spot. On the other hand, it would be a mistake to conclude that the same gene on two separate arrays had different levels of expression just because the control on one array was 10 and on the other array was 30. One solution to this is to increase the lower expressed values to a fixed value when there is abundant expression in the other channel.

These ideas lead to the recommendations in Table 5.1 as a modification of the formula presented in Equation (4.1). In this table FR and BR denote the foreground and background intensities in the red channel and FG and BG denote the corresponding intensities in the green channel. Table 5.1 involves two threshold values λ_{Low} and λ_{High}. The value λ_{Low} represents a threshold below which the signals are in danger of being heavily influenced by additive

Table 5.1. Recommended Filtering for Low Intensity Spots on Dual-label Arrays

Red Signal	Green Signal	Description	Recommended log ratio
$FR - BR < \lambda_{Low}$	$FG - BG < \lambda_{High}$	Red signal too low, Green signal not high enough to be conclusive	EXCLUDE
$FR - BR < \lambda_{High}$	$FG - BG < \lambda_{Low}$	Green signal too low, Red signal not high enough to be conclusive	EXCLUDE
$FR - BR < \lambda_{Low}$	$FG - BG > \lambda_{High}$	Red signal too low, but Green signal conclusively higher than green	$\log_2 \left(\dfrac{\lambda_{Low}}{FG - BG} \right)$
$FR - BR > \lambda_{High}$	$FG - BG < \lambda_{Low}$	Green signal too low, but Red signal conclusively higher than green	$\log_2 \left(\dfrac{FR - BR}{\lambda_{Low}} \right)$
$FR - BR > \lambda_{Low}$	$FG - BG > \lambda_{Low}$	Both Red and Green are high enough to be used directly	$\log_2 \left(\dfrac{FR - BR}{FG - BG} \right)$

noise. The value λ_{High} represents a value above which we are sure we have a strong signal. Values of $\lambda_{Low} = 200$ and $\lambda_{High} = 500$ are reasonable and will result in a fairly conservative selection of well-measured spots.

5.2.5 Large Relative Background Intensity

Although background subtraction helps to adjust for the effect of background luminescence, the effect of the background on the signal may not be strictly additive. If the background is weak relative to the signal, this nonadditivity will have only a minor effect on the final signal value. However, if the observed background is almost as large as the foreground, this nonadditivity, as well as the noise in the background measurement, will heavily influence the signal. Therefore cases in which the intensity of the background is large relative to the foreground should be viewed with some suspicion.

Many of the spots for which the background is large relative to the foreground will also have low background-adjusted signal, and are correctly dealt with in the previous section. It is, however, possible for a spot to have foreground and background of comparable intensity and yet still have a background-adjusted signal greater than the λ_{Low} threshold discussed in the previous section. For example, this would be the case if $FR = 2250$ and $BR = 2000$. Such spots should be excluded from analysis.

There are several ways in which to identify spots as having a large relative background. The simplest is to require that in each channel of a given spot, the ratio of foreground intensity to background intensity is larger than a set threshold. A reasonable threshold to use would be to exclude spots for which the mean foreground was less than 1.5 times that of the median background in either of the channels. Jenssen et al. (2002) describe an adaptive method for establishing the threshold for spot exclusion based on having a subset of the clones printed in duplicate on each array.

A second method is to exclude those spots for which there is a substantial overlap in the distributions of the intensities of the foreground and background pixels. For example, one might exclude spots for which more than 50% of foreground pixels have values less than one standard deviation above the mean of the intensity of the background pixels. This method requires quite specific information about the pixel level data, but some software packages (such as GenePix) produce this percentage automatically.

Brown et al. (2001) provide a formula for the standard deviation of the ratio of background-adjusted mean red intensity to mean green intensity in terms of the variation of intensity among pixels in the foreground region in each channel and the correlation of red and green pixel intensities in the foreground region. Brown et al. recommend that their formula be used for flagging problematic spots. The formula is similar to that derived by Chen et al. (1997); Brown et al. (2001) note that the problematic spots tend to be those for which the correlation of red and green pixel intensities is not sufficiently high.

5.3 Gene Level Quality Control for Two-Color Arrays

Not all probes (clones or oligonucleotides) will perform equally well in evaluating the expression of a given gene. In some cases, a clone supply may be contaminated or may be mislabeled and, in fact, correspond to a different gene altogether. Furthermore, even if the clone is correct, some clones may not hybridize to the sample as well as others. Additionally, there may be technical problems that lead to poor printing of a given probe. At best, measurements from poorly behaving clones are uninformative and including them in the analysis will act to exacerbate the problem of multiple comparisons (see Chapter 7); at worst, they can lead to erroneous conclusions.

Most of the difficulties with poor quality probes will affect the entire print set of arrays. Therefore, most of the tests of poor probe quality should be done by the experimenter over all arrays in the entire print set. Tests of poor hybridization in the reference channel (Section 5.3.1), however, should be performed over all experiments with the same common reference. Tests for exclusion of low variance genes (Section 5.3.3) should include all of the arrays in the experiment.

Most of the tests of gene quality involve making comparisons of gene expression across multiple arrays. In order for such comparisons to be relevant, it is necessary that they be done after normalization (Chapter 6).

5.3.1 Poor Hybridization and Printing

Some probes will not hybridize well to the target RNA. These probes will give very weak signals and are of little value in the analysis. Additionally, it is possible that there will be an error in printing that results in all spots of a given inventory well having poor quality. Either of these problems will result in large numbers of spots printed from a given well being excluded according to the methods of Section 5.2. If spots for a given well are excluded due to poor quality in more than 50% of the samples, then the well is likely to be of little use and should probably be excluded from analysis.

Using a common reference design, it is difficult to evaluate genes that are not expressed in the reference sample. Therefore, those genes that have consistently low signal values in the reference channel should be viewed with suspicion. A reasonable cutpoint is to exclude those genes for which the median background-adjusted spot signal in the reference channel (taken across all arrays including those spots excluded for low signal) is less than 200.

5.3.2 Probe Quality Control Based on Duplicate Spots

If space allows, it is useful to have duplicates of each gene on the array. This can be done either by printing different probes that target a given gene or by printing multiple copies of the same probe. Detection of poor or mislabeled probes is possible by comparing expression levels for the duplicates.

A good metric to use in checking for agreement between probes is mean squared difference between the log ratios. The formula for this metric between spots k_1 and k_2 is

$$\frac{1}{J} \sum_{j=1}^{J} \left(x_{jk_1} - x_{jk_2} \right)^2, \tag{5.1}$$

where x_{jk} represents the log ratio for spot k on array j. If some of the observations were excluded due to weak signal or other reasons, this average can be taken over the nonexcluded samples. A reasonable threshold would be to say that the multiple probes from the same gene disagree if this mean squared difference is greater than 1.0 on the $\log_2$ scale.

If expression levels for replicate probes of an identical clone fail to agree, it is likely that the problem is technical in nature and one of the probes was poorly printed, contaminated, or mislabeled. It then needs to be determined which of the probes is faulty. If there are three or more replicates, then it may be a matter of identifying the outlier. If only duplicates are available, then identifying the faulty one is more complicated. One can examine the signal intensities and background levels of the two spots and look at the correlation between each duplicate and genes on the array with similar biology.

When there are probes printed from different clones of the same gene, then differences in expression level may be biological in nature. Because different clones may come from different regions of the gene, they may hybridize differently to the same transcript. In addition, mutations or deletions of the gene or post-transcriptional modifications may lead to real differences in the abundance of target transcripts for the clones.

Jenssen et al. (2002) describe an adaptive method for establishing the threshold for spot exclusion based on a sufficient number of clones printed in duplicate on each array. The mean squared difference between duplicates is computed for each gene, and averaged over the genes with duplicate spots. This variance is computed as a function of filter thresholds. A threshold level is selected so that 90% of unfiltered duplicate spots on the same array differ by less than twofold.

5.3.3 Low Variance Genes

Although not necessarily of poor quality, probes that have low variance of log ratio expressions across samples are of questionable utility. For such genes, the observed variability is more likely to be due to measurement noise than actual biological variability. Although these such genes are very useful in tasks such as normalization, it may be best to exclude them from analyses that compare samples or groups of samples, or that cluster samples; they are likely to be uninformative and their inclusion can exacerbate the problem of multiple comparisons (see Chapter 7). Also, computations are faster if there are fewer genes involved, particularly computations involving hierarchical clustering of genes. Potentially, there exists a gene or genes that exhibit a very narrow range of variation but whose tiny fluctuations are exquisitely informative of important biological distinctions. Unfortunately, the ability to obtain sufficiently precise measurements for such genes might be beyond the technical capabilities of current microarray technologies.

To screen out genes exhibiting little variation across microarray experiments, sometimes referred to as *nondifferentially expressed* genes, a number of different approaches are used. Probably the most common approach is to set a threshold for fold-change. For example, for each gene take the highest expression measurement for the gene (across the series of arrays) and divide it by the lowest expression measurement for that gene. Any genes for which this fold-change is less than a threshold such as two or fourfold are deleted prior to analysis. A limitation of this approach is that it does not account for the number of microarrays in the experiment or the number of genes that are examined. As either the number of microarrays or the number of genes increases, the number of truly nondifferentially expressed genes that exceed any fixed threshold will increase.

To account for the number of microarrays, one can take a more statistically based approach such as using the ratio of the 95th percentile to the 5th percentile rather than a max/min ratio-based criterion. Taking percentiles removes the dependence of the expected maximum and minimum on the number of microarrays, and it is more robust to the influence of a few extreme observations.

Alternatively, a variance-based criterion can be used. The variance of the log ratios for a gene across multiple samples is calculated, and all of those genes whose variance falls below a particular threshold are excluded. There are several ways to choose a threshold. One could choose an arbitrary number, for example, exclude all genes whose variance is less than 0.5 on a $\log_2$ scale. One could choose a threshold so that a specified percentage of genes is included, for example, include only genes with variance in the top 30th percentile; the choice of percentile will depend on the composition of the genes included on the array. A similar approach is to compute the proportion of the arrays for which the expression level of the gene is at least twofold different from the median for that gene. Genes for which that proportion is too low, say less than 10%, may be excluded.

5.4 Array-Level Quality Control for Two-Color Arrays

An individual array can fail in many ways. Array fabrication defects, problems with RNA extraction, failed labeling reaction, poor hybridization conditions, and faulty scanning can all lead to an array that is of poor overall quality. In general, it is better to discard or redo such arrays rather than to risk polluting the good data available on the other arrays.

One indicator of poor array quality is the number of spots on the array excluded due to poor quality. A certain number of excluded spots is to be expected given the multitude of difficulties that can lead to a spot being poorly measured. Many of the excluded spots will correspond to clones that failed to hybridize in any of the arrays. Even after the poor clones have been removed, it is not unusual to find arrays on which as many as 30% of the spots are excluded due to weak signal or other reasons. However, if the experimenter finds that one of the arrays has an unusually high number of excluded spots, a number well outside the range of the other arrays, then that sample should either be rearrayed or excluded from analysis.

Another indicator of overall array quality is the ratio of the average of the foreground intensities of the spots on the array, and the average of the background intensities of the spots on the array. Higher-quality arrays generally will have relatively large values for this ratio. A value of three or more in both channels can generally be considered a good array, and a ratio less than two in either channel is likely to indicate an array of poor quality.

A third indicator of poor array quality is very low variance of red or green intensities across the spots represented on the array. Generally, there should be a substantial range of intensities for each channel. Assersohn et al. (2002) recommended that if the standard deviation of the $\log_{10}$ channel-specific intensities did not exceed 0.25 (corresponding to a standard deviation of 0.83 for $\log_2$ intensities), then one should suspect the quality of the arrays.

A fourth indicator of array quality is the number of saturated pixels. As mentioned in Section 4.1, photon intensities may reach a range beyond the limits of analogue-to-digital converters. In these cases a signal is reported that is equal to the largest value that can be represented. This necessarily leads to an underestimation of the true output signal. A few spots with saturated pixels are to be expected. However, if significant numbers of spots with saturated pixels are observed (e.g. if more than 2% of the spots on the array have more than half of their pixels saturated), then it may be best to rescan the array with a lower PMT voltage.

One final indicator of array quality is the amount of adjustment required for the array. Data normalization, discussed in Chapter 6, is used to correct for biases between different arrays on the same experiment. If it is found that the observed signals on a given array need to be substantially changed to make the array comparable to the other arrays, it is likely that there is a problem on that array that may not be correctable by normalization. A reasonable criterion would be to be suspicious of any array for which a linear normalization of more than threefold (±1.6 on the $\log_2$ scale) is required. For cases in which the normalization factor varies between genes within an array (location-based or intensity-based normalization) it is reasonable to require that no more than 10% of the points require normalization by more than fourfold (±2 on the $\log_2$ scale).

5.5 Quality Control for GeneChip™ Arrays

The above discussion was directed primarily to two-color cDNA microarrays. Some of the techniques can be applied to Affymetrix arrays, but many are difficult to implement because the measure of expression of a single gene is based on multiple probe pair measurements. Some useful quality control measures are implemented in software such as Affymetrix's Micro Array Suite (MAS), or the dChip[1] software created by Li and Wong to aid in quality control. In this section we describe several of the MAS and dChip quality control measures and make some additional suggestions.

As with two-color arrays, an initial visual inspection of the array image is an important first step. From the visual inspection of the array image one can check the overall quality of the array, check to be sure that the gridding was successful, and identify any obvious anomalies (bright or dark patches, edge effects, debris, etc.). Probe pairs in regions that are contaminated by such anomalies can then be flagged and excluded from the analysis.

---

[1] http://biosun1.harvard.edu/complab/dchip/.

Each gene in a GeneChip^{TM} array is represented by multiple probe pairs, which are scattered across the array, therefore, gene-level quality control for individual arrays is more complex than for cDNA arrays. Fortunately, a number of software packages can assist in this quality control. The algorithm MAS uses will down weight individual outlying probe pairs in forming its signal measurement for a given gene. The dChip software (Li and Wong 2001a) attempts to model the relative sensitivity of different probe pairs with regard to their ability to measure gene expression and then discards as poor quality those probes that do not fit the model.

A number of other quality control indices are available through MAS. MAS report the average background of the array. As with two-color arrays, Affymetrix arrays with high background are more likely to be of poor quality. A reasonable cutoff would be to exclude arrays with a value more than 100. A second measure of array quality is the raw noise score, which is referred to as Q by the MAS software. This is a measure of the variability of the pixel values within a probe cell averaged over all of the probe cells on an array. This value will vary from scanner to scanner, so it is difficult to provide a universal cutpoint. A reasonable approach would be to exclude those arrays that have an unusually high Q-value relative to other arrays that were processed with the same scanner.

Along with a measure of gene expression, the MAS software produces a call as to whether the gene transcript is present or absent in the sample, and provides a p-value for this call. This p-value is based on a Wilcoxon signed-ranked test between the perfect match and the mismatch probe intensities. If most of the perfect match probes have larger intensity than the mismatch probes, then this is an indication that the gene is present. On the other hand, if the distributions of the perfect match and mismatch probes largely overlap, then this would indicate the gene is absent from the sample. Because there may be correlations between probe intensities, the p-value reported is not strictly valid and should not be directly used as a measure of statistical significance. Still, the present/absent call may be a useful tool for screening genes and detecting problems with the array.

Any gene that is absent from the sample should have a true expression of zero. Any fluctuation in the signal of such genes is therefore due to noise rather than any true expression difference. Unlike spots on cDNA arrays that have low expression in both channels, these probe sets are informative because their low signals do represent low gene expression. However, comparing expression levels across multiple arrays in which the gene is absent is not likely to be fruitful. Therefore, if a gene is called absent on almost all of the samples, it may be of little use and should probably not be included in the analysis. Nevertheless, an exception should be made if those few arrays on which the gene is present have a very strong signal. In this case the gene may make a clear distinction between the two sets of arrays (one in which it is clearly present and one in which it is absent) and so should be retained in the analysis.

The number of genes that are declared absent on a given array will clearly depend on the type of tissue being analyzed and the type of array being used. However, if one of the arrays has an unusually large number of absent genes relative to the other arrays in the experiment, then the array may have failed to hybridize well.

In addition, there are several spiked controls (bioB, bioC, bioD, and cre) that are included in the sample as part of the GeneChip^{TM} protocol. BioB is included at a concentration that is close to the level of detection of the array, and so should be indicated as present about 50% of the time. The remaining spiked controls are included at increasingly greater levels of concentration. Therefore, they should all be indicated as present, and also should have increasingly large signal values:

$$\text{Signal(bioB)} < \text{Signal(bioC)} < \text{Signal(bioD)} < \text{Signal(cre)}.$$

If these spiked controls are declared absent by the MAS software, or have values that are not ordered as above, there was either a problem with the hybridization of these controls or a failure to follow the prescribed protocol. In either case, it would probably be best to exclude the array.

As with two-color arrays, the amount of normalization required is an indicator of array quality in GeneChip^{TM} arrays. Unlike two-color arrays, there are several ways in which to choose a baseline against which to normalize a GeneChip^{TM} array; see Section 6.4. For this reason, we cannot suggest an upper limit to the amount of normalization that is acceptable. What is important is that all arrays have approximately the same amount of normalization. If one array has a normalization factor that is more than three times as large as other arrays in the experiment, then the array may be poorly measured.

In the case of GeneChip^{TM} arrays, much of the gene quality control has already been done by Affymetrix. They have done their best to weed out oligonucleotides that have failed to reliably correlate with gene expression. Still, if there are genes for which multiple probe sets are available, it is worthwhile checking to see whether the expressions for the different versions of the gene agree. As with two-color arrays, this can be done by checking the mean squared difference of the signal value for the duplicates; refer to Section 5.3.2 for details.

5.6 Data Imputation

After performing the filtering described previously, there will generally be a large number of missing values in the dataset. If the analyses that are being performed are done on a gene-by-gene basis, then it is best simply to ignore the samples on which the gene has missing values and analyze each gene based solely on samples for which values are present. However, some analyses will be performed using multiple genes. In such analyses, excluding all samples missing any one gene results in few, if any, samples left to analyze. Some of these analyses can be modified to handle missing data, but others may require that the dataset contain no missing values. For such analyses, one could restrict the analysis to only those genes that are present on all samples, but doing so may eliminate important genes that have missing values on only a few of the arrays. Under these circumstances, it may be necessary to impute values to replace missing data. Because imputation involves comparing gene expression across arrays, it should be done after normalization (Chapter 6).

There is a large statistical literature concerned with the problem of missing data imputation. Little and Rubin (2002) give a good overview of general methods of dealing with missing values. We present two relatively simple methods of data imputation that have been applied successfully to microarray data.

The simplest method of imputing missing values is to replace all missing values for a gene with the median value of the observed values for that gene. For two-color arrays, one imputes log ratio values. Median value imputation has the advantage of providing a relatively neutral result for the missing data, and so these imputed values will not heavily influence conclusions drawn from the data. However, inasmuch as there is no biological connection between the sample and the imputed array value, including these imputed values in the analysis will tend to dilute any real effect observed in the other samples. This method may also have the disadvantage of creating a potentially large subset of samples all of which share identical values for a gene. This could cause difficulties for certain analyses that make use of the distribution of a gene's values.

A second method of imputation uses the inherent correlation between expressions of different genes on the array to provide an educated guess as to the correct value for missing genes (Troyanskaya et al. 2001). This method is a variation of K-nearest neighbor prediction and is implemented as follows. Assume that we wish to impute a value for a gene in sample m and let $Y = \{y_1, \ldots, y_J\}$ represent the vector consisting of the normalized log ratios for this gene across all arrays in which its value is present. Let y_m be the missing value we wish to impute. Calculate the mean squared difference (MSD) distance between Y and every other gene X. In this calculation you utilize every sample that is not missing values in either Y or X. Identify the N genes most similar to the gene whose value you need to impute with respect to this distance. For Y_m we impute the weighted average of the expression for these genes on sample m. The weights are the reciprocals of the distances. Troyanskaya et al. (2001) found that a value for N between 10 and 20 worked well for their data. Software for this method is available at http://smi-web.stanford.edu/projects/helix/pubs/impute.

This method has the advantage that it allows the imputed value to be influenced by the biology of the sample and so may be less likely to dilute true effects than the use of the median for the gene. In addition, because the imputed values will differ from sample to sample, this method will not lead to many samples sharing the same values for a gene. Troyanskaya et al. (2001) showed that the imputed values generated by this method are more accurate than using the median when samples are missing at random. Therefore, this method will work well for spots that were excluded due to bubbles, scratches, or other array anomalies that are caused more by the location of genes on the chip rather than signal quality. It is not so clear that this method performs as well when samples are missing due to low signal intensity. If a spot on an array is missing due to low signal, it is likely that many other samples will also be missing values for this same gene that may make it more difficult to identify other genes with similar expression. Furthermore, those genes that share similar expression may also have low signals and be missing for that sample. As a result, the genes that are averaged to form the imputed value may not be very close in expression to the gene for which the value was imputed and may themselves not be of good quality.

6

Array Normalization

6.1 Introduction

Before comparing the gene expression values between arrays, the arrays must be normalized. This step is necessary because there is likely to be an observed intensity imbalance between RNA samples, which will affect all genes. This imbalance has nothing to do with the biology of the samples, but instead occurs for a variety of technical reasons, such as differences in the setting of the PMT voltage, imbalance in the total amount of RNA available in each sample, or differences in the uptake of the dyes. The amount of normalization required will vary from array to array. The objective of normalization is to adjust the gene expression values of all genes on the array so that the genes that are not really differentially expressed have similar values across the arrays. There are two decisions that need to be made: which genes to use as the normalization genes and which normalization algorithm to use.

6.2 Choice of Genes for Normalization

Ideally, we wish to normalize using genes that have similar expression across our samples. If this is not the case, we run the risk of confusing true biological differences in which we are interested with the artifacts we are trying to eliminate by normalization. Several strategies can be used to obtain a set of genes on which to base the normalization.

6.2.1 Biologically Defined Housekeeping Genes

Housekeeping genes are genes that are involved in the essential activities of cell maintenance and survival, but which are not involved in cell function or proliferation. Because all cells need to express these genes to survive, it is reasonable to expect that such genes will be similarly expressed in all samples in the experiment. Therefore, such housekeeping genes make perfect candidates to use in normalization.

Unfortunately, it is often difficult to identify housekeeping genes. In addition, genes that are housekeeping genes for one type of tissue may not be housekeeping genes for a different type. Therefore, unless carefully controlled experiments have been performed demonstrating that the expression of the gene is high and approximately constant for the type of tissue being studied, it cannot be known for sure whether the gene can be appropriately considered a housekeeping gene.

The GeneChip^{TM} arrays contain genes that Affymetrix claims to be housekeeping genes. These genes were tested on a large number of different tissue types and were found to have quite low variability in the tested samples. These are certainly good candidates to use as housekeeping genes, but because it is impossible to test all possible tissue types, there is still no guarantee that the genes will be biologically invariant in every experiment. Therefore, if it is decided to use these housekeeping genes to normalize the data, it is worthwhile checking to be sure that, after normalization, all of these housekeeping genes have low variability across the set of samples used in the experiment.

6.2.2 Spiked Controls

A second method of array normalization is to include in both the reference and the control samples some RNA that is generally not found in either sample, for example, putting some yeast RNA into human samples. By placing the same relative amount of RNA into both samples hybridized to a two-color array, it is possible to create an artificial housekeeping gene that will have equal expression in both channels. If these artificial genes are spotted on the chip, we will be able to detect bias and be sure of the fact that it was not due to biological differences.

The difficulty with this method is that in order for it to provide the correct normalization, it is necessary that the proportion of sample RNA to spiked control be the same in both channels. This implies that the experimenter must be able to determine the actual amount of RNA included in each channel, and then be able to add the foreign RNA proportionally. Doing so may be technically challenging.

The Affymetrix GeneChip^{TM} protocol includes the spiking of control oligonucleotides into each sample. These controls are included to aid in measuring the effectiveness of hybridization and to aid in the gridding of the slide by the image analysis software. There is no fixed relationship between the amount of control used and the amount of available RNA in the sample, therefore these controls should not be used for normalization. Furthermore, the investigator should not be concerned if, even after normalization, the expression of these controls varies from slide to slide.

6.2.3 Normalize Using All Genes

The simplest approach is to use all of the adequately expressed genes for normalization. The underlying assumption for this approach is that the majority of the genes on the array are housekeeping genes. In fact, for the simplest normalization methods we present (Section 6.3, and 6.4), all that is required for a set of normalization genes is that the proportion of genes that are over expressed in a given sample be approximately equal to the proportion of genes that are under expressed. These assumptions will hold for most randomly selected sets of genes. Therefore, this method works well in cases where there are a large number of genes included on the array and when the majority of the genes were not specifically selected to be differentially expressed between the experimental and reference samples. However, if the genes on the array were carefully selected to be genes of specific biological interest that are highly variable across the samples, then it will be necessary to include a separate set of either housekeeping genes or spiked controls to use in normalization.

6.2.4 Identification of Housekeeping Genes Based on Observed Data

There are several techniques for using the observed data to identify housekeeping genes. For two-color arrays, Tseng et al. (2001) recommend designating as housekeeping genes those genes that have similar ranks in the red and green channels. We find that such techniques often choose those genes that are in the center of the distribution of all log ratios on the array. Therefore, the result of normalizing with respect to this subset is virtually identical to the result obtained by normalizing with respect to the complete list of genes. Wang et al. (2002) present an iterative method for selecting normalization factors and simultaneously identifying genes with low variation across the arrays after normalization.

6.3 Normalization Methods for Two-Color Arrays

Normalization of two-color arrays involves determination of the amount by which the genes on the red channel are over- or underexpressed relative to the green channel. This bias will differ for different arrays and, depending on the form of the bias, may vary by gene. Once the size of the bias is estimated, we obtain our final signal value by subtracting this normalization factor from the observed log ratio. Thus the normalized signal value for clone k on array j will be

$$x_{jk} = \log\left(\frac{R_{jk}}{G_{jk}}\right) - C_{jk},$$

where R_{jk} and G_{jk} denote the background-adjusted red and green signals as in Equation (4.1) and C_{jk} is the normalization factor.

There are several ways of calculating C_{jk}. These methods differ in their modeling of the systematic bias to be corrected by normalization. They can be divided into three categories: linear or *global normalization* in which the normalization factor is the same for all genes on the array, *intensity-based normalization* in which the normalization factor used depends on the signal intensity for that spot, and *location-based normalization* in which the normalization factor depends on the location of the spot on the array. Determining which type of normalization method to use requires examining the observed unnormalized log ratios and deciding what kinds of systematic effects are present. The amount of normalization required will vary by array. Therefore each array should be normalized separately. However, the type of normalization used (linear, intensity, location) should be the same for all arrays in the experiment.

6.3.1 Linear or Global Normalization

The simplest method of normalization uses a single normalization factor applied to all genes on the array, but this value varies from array to array. It is called linear normalization because it assumes that the red and green intensities have an approximately linear relationship through the origin for the normalization genes on a given array. The slope of this linear relationship will determine the amount of normalization required, and will become an additive effect on the log scale.

For this normalization method, all genes on a given array will have the same normalization factor. The formula for linear normalization is

$$C_{jk} \equiv C_j = \operatorname*{median}_{i \in S} \left(\log \left(\frac{R_{jk}}{G_{jk}} \right) \right), \tag{6.1}$$

where S is the set of normalization genes. We use the median rather than the mean because it is less likely to be influenced by outlying values. Also, if we are normalizing with respect to all genes, then according to our assumptions regarding the distribution of up-and down-regulated genes (see Section 6.2.3) the center of the distribution of log ratios should consist of those genes that are not differentially expressed between the red and green channels. By using the median, we focus attention on these center genes.

This method works well for most applications. It will be usable even when there are a relatively small number of normalization genes (e.g. 50 to 100 genes), as is often the case when housekeeping genes or spiked controls are used. This method also has the advantage that it is less likely than other methods to over fit the normalization to the data. Other methods in which the normalization varies from gene to gene are more sensitive to changes in the observed expression of individual genes, and so may produce biased results. For this reason, we recommend linear normalization unless there is compelling evidence that a substantial number of arrays in the experiment require a more complicated normalization method.

6.3.2 Intensity-Based Normalization

In some arrays, it appears that the overall magnitude of the spot intensity may have an impact on the relative intensity between the channels. In order to determine if this is the case, it is recommended that the experimenter look at so-called *M-A plots* (Yang et al. 2002a) in which for each array j the quantity

$$M_{jk} = \log\left(\frac{R_{jk}}{G_{jk}}\right)$$

is plotted against the RNA abundance

$$A_{jk} = \frac{1}{2}\left(\log(R_{jk}) + \log(G_{jk})\right)$$

over all normalization genes. In the above equations M_{jk} represents the log ratio of background-adjusted intensities for gene k on array j. A_{jk} represents the average of the red and green channels with regard to background-adjusted intensity for gene k on array j.

If no normalization is required, the spots will appear symmetrically scattered around the horizontal line $M = 0$. If only a linear normalization is required, then the spots will still be scattered around a horizontal line, but the line will be shifted up or down away from 0 by an amount equal to the required normalization. Figure 6.1(a) shows such a plot. If the spots follow a line with nonhorizontal slope, or a nonlinear curve, then it may be necessary to perform a nonlinear intensity normalization. Figure (6-1(b)) shows such a *M-A* plot. In this case, the spots with high intensity (high A values) have a relatively smaller red signal than green signal (negative M values).

The technical cause of this nonlinearity in normalization is not immediately obvious. It may have to do with a component of background luminescence that acts in a nonadditive way with the foreground, or it may have to do with some aspect of signal saturation in the detector. Whatever the cause, the form of the normalization curve can vary markedly between arrays. Therefore it is necessary to fit a separate normalization curve to each array.

If it has been determined that intensity-based normalization is necessary, the next step is to fit a curve to the *M-A* plot for the normalization genes. Locally weighted regression curves (also known as loess curves) are most frequently used, but other smoothing functions such as splines should produce similar results. The lines in Figures 6.1(a) and (b) show the loess normalization curve fitted to the data.

Once the curve is fitted, we define

$$C_{jk} = f_j(A_{jk}),$$

where f_j is the smoothing function fitted to array j, and A_{jk} is the abundance value for clone k on array j.

In order to perform intensity-based normalization, it is necessary that there be normalization genes across all intensity values. Therefore if there are

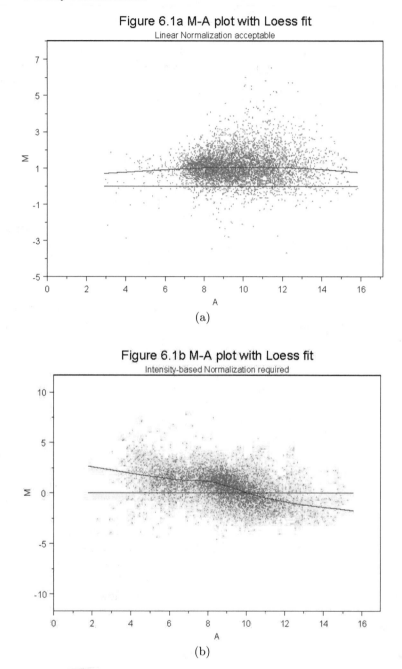

Fig. 6.1. (a) Loess fit to *M-A* plot of array data. Horizontal loess line indicates that constant normalization should be sufficient. (b) Loess fit to *M-A* plot of array data. Clear nonlinearity of loess fit indicates that intensity-based normalization should be used.

only a small number of identified housekeeping or spiked control genes, or if the expressions of these genes do not span the range of expression levels, this normalization method cannot be used. Furthermore, even if all genes are being used to normalize the data, there is the implicit assumption that at each intensity level there are equal numbers of up- and down-regulated genes. If all the high- (or low-) intensity genes share similar biology, it is possible that this assumption could be violated and it would be best to avoid this normalization method.

Another danger of using intensity-based normalization is that at intensities for which there are few spots the normalization could be based on a rather small number of points, and as a result could overfit to those particular values. Thus, by normalizing the data, the experimenter could subtract away exactly the effect he or she was trying to measure if the normalization was performed using all genes.

6.3.3 Location-Based Normalization

Another artifact that is sometimes observed is that the background-subtracted log ratios on the array vary in a predictable manner based on their position on the array. Figure 6.2(a) shows the dependence between log ratios and position on a sample array. The spots along the top and right side of the array appear to be very red, and the lower left corner appears much less red.

One factor that may contribute to location-specific differences in the observed log ratios are differences in the print tips used to create the slide. Because there may be subtle differences in the degree of wear on a print tip, it has been suggested that normalization should be performed separately for each print tip (Yang et al. 2002a).

Figure 6.2(b) shows the median log ratio for each of the 24 grids in the array presented in Figure 6-2a. The lower left grid has a lower median log ratio, as do those around it, and the grids on the top and right side have larger values. Each print tip generates a grid that is located at a separate place on the array. By normalizing with respect to the print tip, we effectively normalize with respect to many of the location differences as well.

To normalize within the grid we apply Equation (6.1) but take the median only over the normalization genes within the grid. Figure 6.2(c) shows the results after location normalization. There is now no clear location dependence for the log ratios.

In order to perform location-based normalization, it is necessary that there be significant numbers of normalization genes within each grid. Therefore this technique will not be applicable for normalizing with respect to a small number of spiked controls or housekeeping genes. In addition, inasmuch as there are fewer genes in each grid than there are on the entire array, there is the same danger of overfitting as there was in the intensity-based normalization.

It is possible that normalizing with respect to the print tip will not completely account for all location effects. Although more complicated methods of

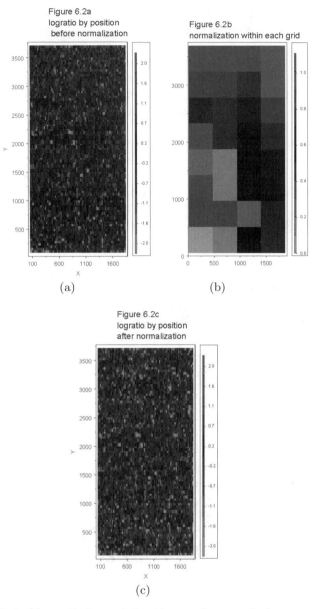

Fig. 6.2. (a) Plot of log ratio for each location on the array before normalization. High enrichment for red along the top and right sides indicates possible need for location-based normalization. (b) Location normalization factors of each grid for array depicted in Figure 6.2(a). (c) Plot of log ratio for each location on the array after location-based normalization. Red and green signals are now dispersed evenly across slide.

location-based normalization exist, many involve the estimation of numerous parameters, and may introduce artifacts by overfitting the data.

6.3.4 Combination Location and Intensity Normalization

If it appears that both location and intensity-based normalization are required, there are two ways to proceed. One possibility is to perform linear normalization separately for each grid and then apply intensity-based normalization to the resulting normalized log ratios on the entire array. Alternatively, the intensity-based normalization can be performed separately within each grid. Yang et al. (2002a) reported that the shape of the loess curves fit to the M-A plots could vary from grid to grid, suggesting that the second alternative might be best. However, the number of available spots within each grid may be relatively low, making the fitted curve dependent on the values of a few points. This is particularly a problem at intensities where data are sparse. Thus there is a danger that true biological variability of an individual spot may be absorbed by the normalization factor and eliminated. Therefore, unless it is very clear that the patterns of the M-A curves vary significantly between grids on the array, we recommend using a single M-A plot fitted to all spots on the array.

6.4 Normalization of GeneChip^{TM} Arrays

As with two-color microarrays, the overall magnitude of the signal for all genes on a given Affymetrix array can vary for technical reasons unrelated to biology. Therefore normalization is necessary. Unlike two-color arrays, there is only a single channel in oligonucleotide arrays. This means that some types of normalization on Affymetrix data must be done between arrays rather than within a single array. Still, many of the same issues that confronted us in two-color array data carry over to Affymetrix data. Both linear normalization methods and intensity-based algorithms have been applied to GeneChip^{TM} arrays. However, location-specific normalization is generally not used. Although location-based intensity imbalances may exist, such imbalances are generally less severe for Affymetrix arrays because the sample is circulated over the surface of probes. Also, because the probe pairs for a gene in Affymetrix arrays are scattered across the array, location-based imbalances will have a smaller effect on the mean differences of individual genes than they did in the case of two-color arrays. As with two-color arrays, the normalization values should be calculated separately for each array, but the normalization method used to calculate these values should be the same for all arrays.

6.4.1 Linear or Global Normalization

As with two-color arrays, the simplest method of normalization is to use a single normalization factor for all genes on the array. This method is used by

Affymetrix's MAS software. This software gives the user the ability either to choose a particular target signal value or to choose a particular baseline array against which to normalize. Based on this choice, the normalization signal log values are calculated as follows.

$$(\text{normalized signal log value})_{jk} = SLV_{jk} - \log_2(sf_j), \quad (6.2)$$

where SLV denotes the signal log value for gene k on array j given by expression (4.3) and sf_j is the scaling factor for array j. The signal value reported by the MAS software is 2 raised to the power of normalized signal log value. Affymetrix software computes the scaling factor as

$$sf_j = \log_2(Sc) - \log_2\left(\text{TrimMean}_k\left(2^{SLV_{jk}}\right)\right), \quad (6.3)$$

where Sc is the target constant used for normalizing all arrays. The "Trim-Mean" notation denotes the mean of the signal values on array j for the housekeeping genes, excluding outliers in the upper and lower 2% of the distribution. Affymetrix computes the trimmed mean on the absolute intensity scale. Because SLV is a $\log_2$ transformed value, the value is raised to the power 2 before taking the trimmed mean. If no housekeeping genes are identified, then the trimmed mean uses the signals for all of the genes on the array. If arrays are normalized to a fixed constant, then Sc is that constant. If a baseline array is chosen for normalization, then Sc is taken as the 2% trimmed mean of the signals for the housekeeping genes on the baseline array.

As we can see from Equations (6.2) and (6.3), changing the target constant or baseline array only results in a different constant being added to all normalized signal log values. Thus it will have no effect on any comparative analyses between arrays provided Sc is the same for all arrays being compared. For this reason, we recommend that if the MAS normalization algorithm is used, the experimenter normalize to the default value of 500 as this will facilitate comparisons between experiments by different investigators.

When considering other normalization methods it should be noted that the MAS software performs its own normalization automatically. Therefore, the signals that are obtainable from the MAS software have already been normalized with their algorithm. Because the MAS normalization is linear, applying a new normalization to signals that were already normalized by MAS will produce the same results as applying the new normalization to the raw signals. Thus, for the purposes of considering alternative normalization methods, the MAS output values can be treated as the raw signal.

6.4.2 Intensity-Based Normalization

Nonlinear intensity-based normalization may also be required in GeneChip^{TM} arrays. To determine whether it is necessary, graphs similar to the $M - A$ plots can be generated. However, rather than comparing different channels from the same array, pairs of arrays are compared. Let X_k denote the normalized signal log value for gene k on one array and Y_k the normalized signal log value for the corresponding gene on a second array; we plot

$$M_k = X_k - Y_k \quad \text{against} \quad A_k = \frac{1}{2}(X_k + Y_k).$$

Because most genes are not expected to vary significantly from array to array, the spots on the plot should be scattered around a horizontal line at 0 if no normalization were needed. If only linear normalization were required, the spots would lie on a horizontal line at a value other than 0. If the spots are scattered around a nonhorizontal line or a nonlinear curve then this will indicate the need for an intensity-based normalization. Unfortunately, because the form of the graph depends on which arrays are paired, a choice must be made as to which array to normalize against. Li and Wong's dCHIP software chooses a single array of medium intensity and then normalizes the probe-level intensities of all other arrays to resemble this one.

Other methods of normalization of Affymetrix data at the probe intensity level are described and compared by Bolstad et al. (2002). They found that a method known as quantile normalization worked best. This method relies on the assumption that even though there may be differences between arrays in the expression of individual probes, the distribution of the expression values should not change dramatically between arrays. Furthemore, they assume that within a single array there is a monotone relationship between the gene expression level and probe value. Therefore they adjust each array in a monotone manner so that all arrays have the identical distribution. The method is as follows. Compute the kth smallest signal value on each array and average them over the arrays. Let $X_{j(k)}$ denote the kth smallest signal on the jth array and let $X_{(k)}$ denote the average over the arrays of their kth smallest signals. Replace $X_{j(k)}$ with $X_{(k)}$ on all of the arrays. Do this for each $k = 1, 2, \ldots$, up to the number of probe sets on the array. Thus, after normalization, all arrays will share the same set of probe signal values, but which probe is associated with which value will vary from array to array depending on the rank ordering of the gene expressions. That is, the 100th smallest value on array 1 will be the same as the 100th smallest value on array 2 but they may represent two different probes. This method of normalization is implemented in the Bioconductor software available at `http://www.bioconductor.org/`.

Even if software that processes probe-level data is not used, an intensity-based normalization can be performed at the signal level. First, a baseline array is chosen to use as a reference; we recommend using an array whose *sf* value is closest to the median of the *sf* values of the arrays being analyzed. The Affymetrix MAS5 software includes the *sf* value for each array as part of the output. The *M-A* plots can then be generated as was done in Section 6.3.2, using the signal for the array being normalized as if it were the test channel and the signal from the baseline array as if it were the reference. If it appears that intensity-dependent normalization is needed, then either quantile normalization or a loess smoother-based normalization can be applied to signal values, again using the baseline array as the reference.

7

Class Comparison

7.1 Introduction

One of the most important goals in microarray studies is to identify genes that are differentially expressed between prespecified classes. Identifying differentially expressed genes with known functions can lead to a better understanding of the biological differences between the classes. Identifying differentially expressed genes with unknown functions can lead to a better understanding of the functions of those genes. The goal of this chapter is different from that of Chapter 9; the goal there is to create classes of specimens for which gene expression is different. *Class comparison* methods are *supervised* in the sense that they utilize the information of which specimens belong to which classes. This is in contrast to methods such as cluster analysis discussed in Chapter 9 which utilize only the expression profiles and are *unsupervised* by any information about class membership.

We begin in Section 7.2 by examining whether a particular gene is differentially expressed between classes. This provides the statistical background for the more realistic problems involving thousands of genes addressed in the remainder of the chapter. Section 7.3 describes how to identify which genes are differentially expressed while controlling for the large number of genes being examined. Section 7.4 describes some methods of analysis of experiments when there are very few specimens in each class available for microarray analysis. Section 7.5 presents global tests of whether there are class differences in gene expression without trying to identify which genes are differentially expressed. Section 7.6 addresses the special situation in which there is only one specimen in each class. A natural generalization of class comparison is to ask whether gene expression is associated with a continuous characteristic or a survival time for the individual from whom the specimen was obtained; this is discussed in Sections 7.7 and 7.8, respectively. Section 7.9 ends the chapter with a discussion of statistical models for analysis of nonreference designs for two-color array experiments.

7.2 Examining Whether a Single Gene is Differentially Expressed Between Classes

We begin by considering the case of two classes, in which case we wish to discover whether a gene has higher expression in one class as compared to the other. As discussed in chapter 4, analyses of expression data typically use logarithmically transformed levels; we use logarithms base 2 for most of our analyses. Suppose one has available J_1 specimens from class 1 and J_2 specimens from class 2. Consider a particular gene, with (transformed) expressions in class 1 given by $x_{11}, x_{12}, \ldots, x_{1J_1}$ and in class 2 given by $x_{21}, x_{22}, \ldots, x_{2J_2}$. One can summarize the average expressions in classes 1 and 2 by the means of the class 1 and class 2 values, $\bar{x}_1$ and $\bar{x}_2$. If $\bar{x}_1$ is larger (smaller) than $\bar{x}_2$, this would suggest that gene is expressed more (less) in class 1 than class 2. There are several things to note about this type of comparison. First, this comparison makes sense even if each expression value is relative to a reference standard (as would generally be the case for cDNA arrays), provided that the same reference standard is used for the specimens in both classes. Second, assuming that the processing of the microarrays is done in the same manner for both classes of specimens, one does not need to be too concerned about sources of systematic bias that are present in the microarrays of both classes; these biases will tend to cancel out when comparing the expressions between classes. For example, with cDNA arrays if the reference specimen is labeled consistently with say, Cy3, then there may be gene-specific dye bias not removed by normalization, but it will not be of concern in comparing the classes. It would only be of concern if we wished to compare either class to the internal reference. Third, only one microarray per specimen is required. If there are replicate arrays on a specimen, we recommend averaging the log expression values to form a single x_{ij} to be used for that specimen, or choosing the array with the best quality; see Chapter 5. Issues concerning whether to design a study with replicate arrays are discussed in Sections 3.4 and 3.7.

Because it is unlikely that the mean expression levels $\bar{x}_1$ and $\bar{x}_2$ will be exactly equal, how does one know that any difference observed between $\bar{x}_1$ and $\bar{x}_2$ is not due to chance? Clearly, a larger rather than smaller difference between $\bar{x}_1$ and $\bar{x}_2$ suggests that the difference is not due to chance. But how large a difference is required? One possibility would be to choose a certain fold difference, for example a twofold difference that corresponds to $|\bar{x}_1 - \bar{x}_2| \geq 1$ when base 2 logarithmic transformations are used. This was the approach used by Lee et al. (1999) when comparing gene expression in 5-month versus 30-month-old mice. A problem with this approach is that it can lead to a high probability of declaring that a gene is differentially expressed when it truly is not (Miller et al. 2001). The approaches described in this section use elementary statistical methods to guard against such chance findings; readers with a statistical background may wish to skip all but the examples in the remainder of this section.

7.2.1 t-Test

In order to guard against chance findings, one must characterize what one means by chance. One notion is as follows. There is a very large population of class 1 and class 2 specimens, and the distributions of the expressions of the class 1 and class 2 specimens are the same in the population. This is referred to as the *null hypothesis*. The J_1 class 1 specimens and J_2 class 2 specimens under investigation are assumed to be (completely) random samples from the class 1 and class 2 specimens, respectively. Statistical theory allows one to estimate the probability that one would see a difference as large as observed. There are different methods to do this. The most commonly used involves a two-sample t-*statistic*,

$$t = \frac{\bar{x}_1 - \bar{x}_2}{\sqrt{s_p^2 \left(\frac{1}{J_1} + \frac{1}{J_2} \right)}}, \tag{7.1}$$

where

$$s_p^2 = \frac{(J_1 - 1) s_1^2 + (J_2 - 1) s_2^2}{J_1 + J_2 - 2}$$

and for $i = 1, 2$,

$$s_i^2 = \frac{1}{J_i - 1} \sum_{j=1}^{J_i} (x_{ij} - \bar{x}_i)^2.$$

The *variance* estimator s_p^2 estimates the (pooled) within-class variability of the gene expressions; its square root is known as the within-class *standard deviation*. An alternative t-statistic uses $\sqrt{s_1^2/J_1 + s_2^2/J_2}$ in the denominator of (7.1). This alternative t-statistic is referred to as the t-statistic using the *separate-variance* formula, whereas (7.1) is referred to as the t-statistic using the *pooled-variance* formula.

One interpretation of the t-statistic is that it is the ratio of between-class to within-class variability of the gene expression. Another interpretation is that the denominator of the statistic is an estimator of the variability of $\bar{x}_1 - \bar{x}_2$ one would see if one repeatedly sampled J_1 class 1 and J_2 class 2 specimens from the very large population. With either interpretation, large positive or negative values of the t-statistic suggest that $\bar{x}_1$ and $\bar{x}_2$ are differing more than by just chance. The t-statistic is converted to a probability, known as a *p-value*, which represents the probability that one would observe under the null hypothesis a t-statistic as large or larger (in absolute value) than the t-statistic calculated from the observed data. For example, one would observe p-values less than 0.01 under the null hypothesis only 1% of the time. The p-value is also sometimes referred to as the *statistical significance* of the data (with respect to the null hypothesis) obtained from a t-test of the null hypothesis. All of our hypotheses tests and p-values will be *two-sided*, representing the fact that we are interested in either class having more expression than the other.

Example 7.1 (Differences in prostate cancer versus benign prostatic hyperplasia (BPH) gene expression for clone 139331 in the Luo Prostate Cancer dataset). The data are from cDNA microarrays done on 16 prostate cancer specimens and 9 BPH specimens; see Appendix B for details. The gene expressions for clone 139331 for 9 prostate cancer specimens and 8 BPH specimens with available data for this clone are displayed in Figure 7.1. We note that

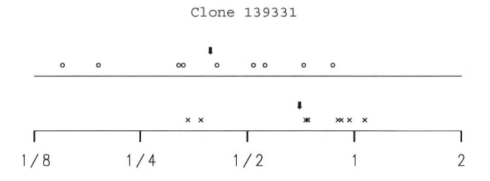

Fig. 7.1. Gene expression relative to the reference sample for clone 139331 for 9 prostate cancer specimens (circle) and 8 BPH (x). Geometric mean expression levels are designated with arrows. (Data are from the Luo Prostate Cancer Dataset.)

the expression levels are on average lower for the prostate specimens than the BPH specimens, with geometric means being 0.39 and 0.70, respectively. (A geometric mean can be defined as 2 raised to the power of the arithmetic mean of the logarithmically (base 2) transformed values.) The p-value from the t-test is $p = .038$. If this had been the only clone studied, then this p-value would suggest that the differences seen in the distributions in Figure 7.1 are not due to chance. However, inasmuch as thousands of clones were examined, this conclusion might be unwarranted; see Example 7.4.

7.2.2 Permutation Tests

The calculation of the p-value from the t-statistic implicitly assumes that the statistical distribution of the numerator of (7.1) is approximately normal (i.e., Gaussian). Because the normal distribution can be completely characterized by its mean and standard deviation parameters, t-tests are examples of what are known as *parametric tests*. The normal distribution approximation may not be good if one is interested in extremely small p-values (as will sometimes be the case in Section 7.3). An alternative approach to estimating p-values that does not depend on approximate normal distributions is via *permutation tests.* One example of a permutation test, the *permutation t-test*, is given as follows. First, the t-statistic is calculated using (7.1). Then the class labels of the $J_1 + J_2$ specimens are randomly permuted, so that a random J_1 of the specimens are temporarily labeled as class 1, and the remaining J_2 specimens are labeled as class 2. Using these temporary labels, the t-statistic (7.1) is calculated, say, t^*. The labels are permuted many times with a calculation of t^* each time. The (two-sided) p-value from the permutation t-test is estimated by

$$p\text{-value} = \frac{1 + \# \text{ of random permutations where } |t^*| \geq |t|}{1 + \# \text{ of random permutations}}. \qquad (7.2)$$

With small sample sizes or in some special cases, one can actually enumerate all

$$\binom{J_1 + J_2}{J_1} \equiv \frac{(J_1 + J_2)!}{(J_1! J_2!)}$$

permutations and use

$$p\text{-value} = \frac{\# \text{ of permutations where } |t^*| \geq |t|}{\binom{J_1 + J_2}{J_1}} \qquad (7.3)$$

rather than the estimator (7.2). (The symbol $J!$ means $J \times (J-1) \times (J-2) \times \cdots \times 2 \times 1$.) A schematic example of the calculation using hypothetical data is given in Figure 7.2: With 5 observations in one class and 4 in the other, there are a total of $\binom{9}{5} = 126$ possible permutations for the data. For the data shown, the absolute value of the t-statistic is 3.64 which is less than or equal to 3 of the permuted dataset absolute t-statistics; the t-statistics corresponding to these 3 datasets are shown in bold type. (Note that the original dataset is considered to be one of the permuted datasets for this calculation.) The permutation p-value is therefore $3/126 = .024$.

Example 7.2 (Permutation t-test for differences in gene expression for clone 139331 in the Luo prostate dataset.). This is a continuation of Example 7.1. The gene expressions for clone 139331 for 9 prostate cancer specimens and 8 BPH specimens with available data for this clone are displayed in Figure 7.1. Because there were missing data in this example (7 prostate cancer specimens and 1 BPH specimen), there are two different ways to permute the class labels. One possibility is to ignore the missing data and randomly assign 16 of the original specimens to be class 1 and the remainder to be class 2. Note that, if done in this way, the numbers of class 1 specimens with available data can change from permutation to permutation. The other possibility is to restrict the permutations to the non-missing specimens and to randomly assign 9 of the 17 specimens with non-missing data to be class 1 and the remainder of the 17 to be class 2. In this case, each permuted dataset will have exactly 9 class 1 specimens. We recommend using the first method, that is, permuting the class labels for all the specimens regardless of whether expression data

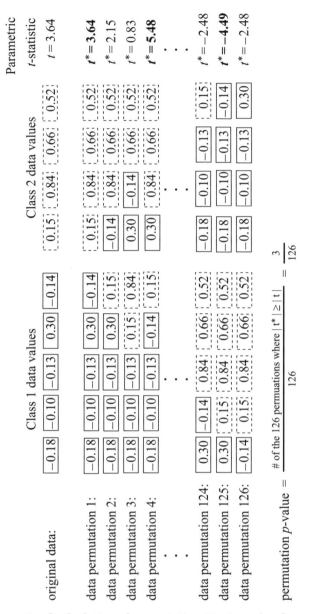

Fig. 7.2. Schematic of calculation of permutation *t*-test *p*-value for unpaired two-class comparison (hypothetical data with five observations in class 1 and four observations in class 2).

are available for this clone for the specimen. (This method has the practical advantage of only having to look at one set of permutations when multiple genes with different patterns of missing data are examined as in Section 7.3.) In the present example, there are $\binom{25}{16}$ possible permutations, of which 9,999 are randomly chosen. Of these random permutations, 378 had $|t^*| \geq |t|$. Therefore the permutation p-value is 0.0379, almost identical in this case to the parametric t-test p-value.

An alternative permutation test to the permutation t-test is the *Wilcoxon rank-sum test* (Hollander and Wolfe 1999). The original $J_1 + J_2$ expression levels are replaced with their ranks. That is, the largest x value of the combined set of $J_1 + J_2$ values is given the value 1, the second largest, the value 2, and this ranking is continued until the smallest is given the value $J_1 + J_2$. The sum of the ranks for only those observations in class 1 is then calculated. This sum is compared to specially constructed tabled values to calculate the p-value (large or small values of the sum indicate class differences). The p-value from the Wilcoxon rank-sum test is the same as would be obtained by performing the permutation t-test on the ranks of the data. The advantages of the Wilcoxon rank-sum test over the permutation t-test are that the permutations do not have to be constructed (because the p-value depends only on the rank sum and J_1 and J_2) and, inasmuch as ranks are used, the rank-sum test will be relatively insensitive to extremely large or small values. The use of the ranks, however, makes the rank-sum test less sensitive to some real differences in the data. Because of this disadvantage and because with modern computing the calculation of the permutations is not difficult, we recommend using the permutation t-test.

When there are a very small number of specimens available from each class, the inferences available from any of the permutation tests are limited in the sense that the obtainable p-values cannot be very small. For example, with 3 specimens in one class and 2 in the other, the smallest obtainable p-value is 0.10 because there are only 10 possible permutations (some definitions of two-sided p-values for permutation tests would consider the two-sided p-value 0.20). The p-values from parametric t-tests can be small even with very small numbers of specimens, but these tests may not be very efficient in detecting true class differences in this situation because the estimates of the within-class variability may be poor. As there are more options for addressing the problem of small numbers of specimens when multiple genes are being considered, we postpone further discussion of this topic to Section 7.4.

7.2.3 More Than Two Classes

For some applications, there will be more than two classes of specimens to compare. For example, specimens may be available from three different histologic subtypes of cancer. The question addressed here is whether there are any differences in the gene expression among the classes. In particular, the null hypothesis is that the distribution of gene expression is the same for all the classes. The *alternative hypothesis* is that at least one of the classes has a distribution of gene expression that is different from the other classes. The statistic analogous to the *t*-statistic appropriate for more than 2 classes is the *F-statistic* (in obvious notation):

$$F = \frac{[J_1(\bar{x}_1 - \bar{x})^2 + J_2(\bar{x}_2 - \bar{x})^2 + \cdots + J_I(\bar{x}_I - \bar{x})^2]/(I - 1)}{s_p^2},$$

where

$$s_p^2 = \frac{1}{J_1 + J_2 + \cdots + J_I - I} \sum_{i=1}^{I} \sum_{j=1}^{J_i} (x_{ij} - \bar{x}_i)^2$$

and

$$\bar{x} = \frac{1}{J_1 + J_2 + \cdots + J_I} \sum_{i=1}^{I} \sum_{j=1}^{J_i} x_{ij}$$

are estimators of the within-class variability and overall mean of the gene expression. Because the *F*-statistic is the ratio of between-class to within-class variability of the gene expression, large values of the statistic suggest observed differences in mean expression among the classes are not due to chance. The *F*-statistic is converted into a *p*-value, which is approximately correct provided that the within-class means $\bar{x}_i$ are approximately normally distributed. For $I = 2$, the *p*-value obtained from the *F*-statistic is identical to the *p*-value obtained from the pooled-variance *t*-statistic.

Analogously to the permutation *t*-test, one can calculate the *p*-value for the *permutation F-test*: The class labels are randomly permuted so that J_1 of the specimens are temporarily labeled class 1, J_2 of the remaining specimens are temporarily labeled class 2, and so on. The numerator of the *F*-statistic is calculated on this temporary dataset. There are $(J_1 + J_2 + \cdots + J_K)!/(J_1!J_2!\ldots J_K!)$ different permuted datasets possible, and they are randomly sampled or completely enumerated if there are not too many of them. Then formulas analogous to (7.2) or (7.3) are used to calculate the *p*-value. Alternatively, the ranks of the *x* values can be used in the permutation analysis, yielding the *Kruskal–Wallis test* (Hollander and Wolfe 1999).

The inference available from a small *p*-value from the analyses just described is somewhat limited: the distributions of expressions from the different classes are not all the same. In many applications, one will be interested in which classes are different from which other classes for the gene expression, not just that there is some difference in the classes. One can follow the calculation of the *p*-value from the *F*-statistic with *post hoc comparisons* to assess which classes have different expression levels (Snedecor and Cochran, 1989). However, a simpler approach, which also generalizes more easily to the situation of testing many genes with permutation tests discussed in Section

7.3, is to compare classes two at a time. For example, with three classes, one could compare (using the methods previously described for two classes) class 1 versus class 2, class 1 versus class 3, and class 2 versus class 3.

There are two situations in which this pairwise analysis approach may not be advisable. The first is when there are very small numbers of specimens in each class. In this situation, there may be more of a possibility of detecting true differences in expression among the classes using a single test than being able to detect a difference between any two given classes. This situation may arise when there are many classes and one is interested in whether there is any association of class and expression at all; for example the classes may represent many different timepoints (after a manipulation) at which specimens of a cell line are taken for microarray analysis. The other situation in which pairwise analysis may not be appropriate is when the classes are naturally ordered, for example specimens from normal tissue (class 1), benign tumor tissue (class 2), and malignant tumor tissue (class 3). In this situation one might expect the gene expression, if not the same in the classes, to be ordered, for example most-less-least or least-more-most. In this case, a test that takes into account the ordering of the classes would be more appropriate than either the F-test or all pairwise tests. The *Jonckheere test* is a generalization of the Wilcoxon rank-sum test for this circumstance (Hollander and Wolfe 1999). Another approach treats the class indices (e.g., 1,2,3) as an independent variable in a regression model; see Section 7.7.

7.2.4 Paired-Specimen Data

Sometimes the specimens available for analysis are paired by some characteristic, with one specimen of each pair belonging to class 1 and the other specimen belonging to class 2. If, as is usually the case, the gene expression of specimens within a pair is expected to be more alike than the gene expression from specimens in different pairs (except for the class differences), then the analysis should incorporate the pairing. Let (x_{11}, x_{21}), (x_{12}, x_{22}), ..., (x_{1J}, x_{2J}) be the J pairs of (log-transformed) expressions, where the first member of each pair is from class 1, and the second member is from class 2. The analogous statistic to the two-sample t-statistic is the *paired t-statistic*

$$t = \frac{\bar{x}_1 - \bar{x}_2}{\sqrt{s_d^2/J}}, \qquad (7.4)$$

where

$$s_d^2 = \frac{1}{J-1} \sum_{j=1}^{J} \left[(x_{1j} - x_{2j}) - (\bar{x}_1 - \bar{x}_2) \right]^2.$$

Large absolute values of the statistic suggest any observed differences between the two classes are not due to chance, and the paired t-statistic can be converted to a p-value to quantify this. Because paired data superficially look like unpaired data with sample sizes of J in each class, it is important when doing the analysis to specify paired data when using a computer program that accommodates both paired and unpaired data.

The analogous test to the (two-sample) permutation t-test is the *permutation paired t-test*. The formula for the p-value is identical to (7.2) with the important exception that the permutations used respect the pairing of the data. That is, a permutation of the dataset represents a relabeling of the class 1 and class 2 labels within each pair of specimens; each pair will always consist of the same two numbers as in the original dataset, but the labeling of those two numbers as belonging to class 1 versus class 2 will be permuted. Thus there are 2^J possible permuted datasets that can be randomly sampled. If J is small, then it is reasonable to evaluate the t-statistic on all the permuted datasets and use the analogous formula to (7.3) to calculate the p-value:

$$p\text{-value} = \frac{\#\text{ of permutations where } |t^*| \geq |t|}{2^J}. \tag{7.5}$$

The *Wilcoxon signed-rank test* (Hollander and Wolfe 1999) is another permutation test for paired data, which uses the ranks of the differences between the expression levels from the paired specimens.

Example 7.3 (Differences in pre and postchemotherapy gene expression for clone AA133129 in the Perou dataset). The data are from cDNA microarrays performed on 20 matched pairs of breast cancer specimens obtained before and after chemotherapy; see Appendix B for details. As compared to the reference sample, the geometric mean for the prechemotherapy expression levels is 0.68, and for the postchemotherapy is 1.37. Thus there is an average twofold increase in expression associated with the chemotherapy. Figure 7.3 shows for each matched pair the ratio of the postchemotherapy expression to the prechemotherapy expression. We see that this ratio is greater than 1 for 19 of the 20 matched pairs. Applying the paired t-test formula (7.4) on the

Clone AA133129

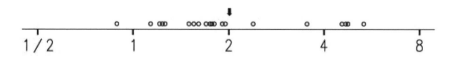

Fig. 7.3. Ratio of postchemotherapy to prechemotherapy gene expression for clone AA133129 for 20 matched pairs of breast cancer specimens. Geometric mean of the ratio is designated with an arrow. (Data are from Perou Dataset.)

logarithms of the expression data, the p-value obtained is 1.19×10^{-5}. The resulting difference is highly statistically significant with such a small p-value. However, as mentioned previously, the exact value of such a low p-value may not be accurate with a parametric test. Using a permutation test with a random selection of permutations will also yield a small p-value, but to get an accurate estimate with a p-value this small would require an inordinately large number of random permutations. However, because of the extreme nature of the pre and post differences for this particular example, one can calculate (7.5) and find the permutation paired t-test p-value is $4/2^{20} = 3.81 \times 10^{-6}$ (details not shown).

7.3 Identifying Which Genes Are Differentially Expressed Between Classes

In Section 7.2 we considered the case of one gene and asked whether it was differentially expressed between classes. In this section we consider the more realistic situation in which there are thousands of genes and we wish to identify which, if any, are differentially expressed between classes. One might consider applying the methods of Section 7.2 to each gene, one gene at a time, and identifying all genes with p-values less than 0.05. The problem with this approach is that under the null hypothesis that no genes are differentially expressed, one will still find on average 5% of the genes with p-values less than .05. For example, with 10,000 genes, one will find on average 500 genes that have p-values less than 0.05, that is, 500 false positives. This is known as a *multiple comparisons problem.* One approach to this problem would be to repeat the study with new sets of specimens from each class and focus on only the genes found to be differentially expressed in the first study. However, using this approach with p-values less than 0.05, one would still find 25 $(= .05 \times 500)$ false positives at the end of the second study. The problem of multiple comparisons is somewhat mitigated if the investigator has a prespecified set of a small number of genes to be studied. It is important that this set of genes be explicitly stated before the experiment is conducted and not chosen on the basis of the gene expression results. Otherwise, all of the genes on the array must be considered toward the multiple comparisons.

In this section we discuss various approaches to control the number of false positives in one study when examining many genes for differential expression. These approaches are of three types: one type controls for no false positives, another type allows some, but not too many, false positives, and still another keeps low the proportion of identified genes that are false positives. We consider these approaches in turn.

7.3.1 Controlling for No False Positives

Most often, one is willing to allow for a small number of false positives as described in Sections 7.3.2 and 7.3.3. In that case, this section can be viewed as an introduction to the methods described in those sections.

7.3.1.1 Bonferroni Methods

Suppose one desired an identification procedure such that one could be 95% confident that all of the genes identified as being differentially expressed were truly differentially expressed, that is, no false positives. (This is sometimes referred to as control of the *familywise error* or *experimentwise error*.) A very simple procedure to do this is as follows. Obtain the p-values for testing class differences for one gene at a time. If K genes are examined, then multiply each of the K p-values by K to obtain the *Bonferroni-adjusted p-values*. Identify as being significantly differentially expressed those genes whose Bonferroni-adjusted p-values are less than .05. (To distinguish these p-values adjusted for multiple comparisons from those calculated on a single gene with no adjustments, we refer to the latter as *unadjusted univariate p-values*.) Note that because the Bonferroni-adjustment depends on the number of genes being examined, it is more difficult to identify truly differentially expressed genes when thousands of genes are being examined. (There is a subtlety here in what constitutes examining a gene. Clearly, if one performs a t-test and calculates a p-value for differential expression for a gene, then that gene has been examined. But what if one eliminates from consideration genes whose data are mostly missing or whose variability over all the specimens (regardless of class) is less than some constant (as described in Section 5.3.3). Have these genes been examined? Although the answer is partly, we would not consider these genes examined for the purposes of the Bonferroni adjustment because their differential class expression was not checked.)

Example 7.4 (Genes showing differential expression in prostate cancer versus. BPH in the Luo Prostate Cancer dataset: Bonferroni adjustment). The data are from cDNA microarrays performed on 16 prostate cancer specimens and 9 BPH specimens; see Appendix B for details. In Example 7.1, we considered differential expressions for clone 139331, and obtained a p-value of 0.038 from a t-test. This is one of 6500 clones on the microarray. If we restrict attention to clones for which there were data from at least 3 prostate cancer specimens and 3 BPH specimens, this reduces the number of analyzed clones to 5854. The Bonferroni-adjusted p-value for clone 139331 is $p = 0.038 \times 5854 > 1$, so with control for the multiple comparisons there is no evidence that this gene is differentially expressed. Forty-seven genes have unadjusted p-values $< .05/5854 = 8.54 \times 10^{-6}$, so their Bonferroni-adjusted p-values are < 0.05.

Example 7.5 (Differences in pre- and postchemotherapy gene expression in the Perou dataset: Bonferroni adjustment). The data are from cDNA microarrays performed on 20 matched pairs of breast cancer specimens obtained before and after chemotherapy; see Appendix B for details. Genes for which data were missing from more than half of the 20 paired specimens were eliminated from consideration. This left 8029 genes for analysis. In Example 7.3, we noted that the unadjusted univariate p-value for clone AA133129 was 1.19×10^{-5} from the parametric paired t-test. This corresponds to a Bonferroni-adjusted p-value of 0.096. Although this gene does not have an adjusted p-value < 0.05, there are 11 genes that do have adjusted p-values < 0.05 based on the parametric paired t-test.

There are two problems with the Bonferroni approach. The first is that in order to be able to decide whether the adjusted p-value is less than a reasonably small number (e.g., 0.05), one has to be able to determine whether the unadjusted univariate p-value is less than an extremely small number (e.g., 0.000005). This is problematic when using either parametric t-tests or permutation tests: p-values from parametric t-tests as described in Section 7.2 are not very accurate in this low range unless the data are exactly normally distributed (an unlikely situation) or the number of specimens (sample size) is very large (another unlikely situation). Although the p-values from the permutation t-tests are valid no matter how small, one cannot obtain extremely small p-values using them with small sample sizes. For example, with 8 specimens in one class and 10 in the other, the smallest possible obtainable unadjusted p-value is 0.00002285 because there are 43,758 possible permutations of which one yields the most extreme t-statistic. Therefore the smallest Bonferroni-adjusted p-value obtainable with 10,000 genes is 0.2285 using a permutation t-test.

The other problem with the Bonferroni approach is that it is conservative in the sense that other approaches may be able to identify more genes that are truly differentially expressed. If the expression data from the different genes were not correlated, this conservative behavior would be minimal. However, because one would expect correlation among the expression levels, the Bonferroni approach can be quite conservative.

Various simple improvements to make the Bonferroni procedure less conservative are based on stepping through the genes and using different adjustments for each one (Holm 1979; Hochberg 1988). Unfortunately, these methods offer little benefit in the situation here where only a small percentage of the genes are differentially expressed.

7.3.1.2 Multivariate Permutation Methods

Fortunately, there are multivariate permutation approaches that avoid the first problem with the Bonferroni approach and are less conservative as well. One such approach first calculates the unadjusted univariate p-values for each gene using a parametric approach, for example, based on a parametric two-sample t-statistic (7.1). Let $p_1, p_2, \ldots, p_K$ be these p-values. The specimen labels are then permuted many times, with the method of permutation depending on the structure of the experiment. Recall from Section 7.2 that with an (unpaired) two-class comparison with J_1 specimens in one class and J_2 specimens in the other, there are $\binom{J_1+J_2}{J_1}$ permutations, whereas for a paired two-class comparison with J pairs of specimens, there are 2^J permutations. For each permuted dataset, the unadjusted univariate p-values are calculated, $p_1^*, p_2^*, \ldots, p_K^*$, and then ordered, $p_{(1)}^* \leq p_{(2)}^* \leq \cdots \leq p_{(K)}^*$. For example, if the tenth gene produces the third smallest p-value, then $p_{(3)}^* = p_{10}^*$. The p-value for the kth gene adjusted for multiple comparisons is then given by

$$\text{adjusted } p\text{-value}_k = \frac{1 + \# \text{ of random permutations where } p_{(1)}^* \leq p_k}{1 + \# \text{ of random permutations}} \quad (7.6)$$

or where it is possible to enumerate all permutations,

$$\text{adjusted } p\text{-value}_k = \frac{\# \text{ of permutations where } p_{(1)}^* \leq p_k}{\# \text{ of all possible permutations}}. \quad (7.7)$$

The idea behind this approach is that to decide whether an unadjusted p-value is small enough to be real, one needs a reference distribution of the smallest p-value of K p-values under the null hypothesis. This reference distribution is provided by the permutation distribution of $p_{(1)}^*$. A schematic example of the method to identify differentially expressed genes in order to have 95% confidence that there are no false positives is given in Figure 7.4. Identification of such genes is equivalent to finding genes whose adjusted p-values are $\leq .05$. Note that to identify such genes, one computationally does not actually have to calculate the adjusted p-value for each gene. Operationally, the procedure reduces to finding the sixth smallest of the $126p_{(1)}^*$ ($6/126 < .05 < 7/126$) and identifying all genes whose univariate p-values are less than or equal to this value.

This approach implicitly uses the correlation structure of the data and therefore will be less conservative than the Bonferroni approach. In addition, inasmuch as it is generating the reference distribution of the quantity of interest directly from the permutations, it does not require either a normal distribution assumption or the calculation of extremely small permutation p-values. An early application of multivariate permutation methods to gene expression data is given by Callow et al. (2000).

Example 7.6 (Genes showing differential expression in pre- and postchemotherapy gene expression in the Perou dataset: multivariate permutation adjustment). This is a continuation of Example 7.5. A sample of 100,000 permutations from 2^{20} possible permutations was used. Seventeen genes were identified as having differential expressions with adjusted p-values < 0.05. (These 17 genes are the 17 genes with the smallest unadjusted univariate p-values, and therefore contain the 11 genes identified by the Bonferroni procedure.) A

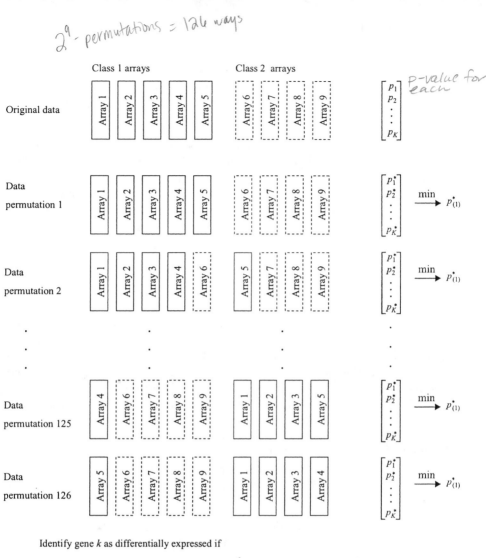

Fig. 7.4. Schematic of method to identify differentially expressed genes for the two-class comparison (five observations in class 1 and four observations in class 2) in order to have 95% confidence that there are no false positives. The univariate p-values $p_1, \ldots, p_K$ correspond to two-sample t-statistics for the K genes on the microarray.

cluster analysis of these data did not suggest pre- and postchemotherapy differential expression (Perou et al. 2000), which shows the importance of using an appropriate statistical method for the goal at hand (Korn et al. 2002).

The multivariate permutation method can be made slightly less conservative by considering a stepwise modification; see Westfall and Young (1993, pp. 113–121) for a complete description. For the present application in which we expect that only a small percentage of a large number of genes will be identified as differentially expressed, this modification will have only a trivial effect on the adjusted p-values.

7.3.2 Controlling the Number of False Positives

The criterion of being confident that there are no false positives among the genes identified as being differentially expressed is generally too stringent. After all, genes identified through a microarray analysis would typically be studied further, resulting in later elimination of the false positives. However, with no control for the multiple comparisons, one could easily falsely identify hundreds of genes, a number too large for efficient further study. This suggests using methods that allow for some, but not too many, false positives. One such method is to use a cutoff for the unadjusted p-values that is lower than the conventional 0.05, but not as low as would be implied by the Bonferroni approach. For example, if one identified all genes with univariate unadjusted p-values < 0.001 as being differentially expressed, then one would have on average $0.001 \times K$ false positives. With $K = 10,000$, this would be 10 false positives. Note that although a p-value of .001 is small, it is not extremely small so that the problems associated with using the Bonferroni approach to control for no errors do not arise.

Example 7.7 (Genes showing differential expression in pre- and postchemotherapy gene expression in the Perou dataset: allowing for some false positives). This is a continuation of Example 7.6. With 8029 genes analyzed, if we identify as differentially expressed all genes with unadjusted p-values < 0.001, we expect on average 8 false positives. There are 68 genes that are identified using this criterion.

A potential problem with this simple approach is that although it controls for the number of false positives on average, for any given analysis the actual number of false positives may vary around this average. If this is of concern, the following more complex approach, which is similar to the multivariate permutation approach used to control for no errors, can be used (Korn et al. 2003). Suppose one wanted to be confident that there were $< U$ false positives. Set the *adjusted p-value* for the genes associated with the U smallest p-values $(p_{(1)}, p_{(2)}, \ldots, p_{(U)})$ to be zero. For the other genes, the adjusted p-value for the kth gene is given by the following formula based on permutations of the specimen labels as described previously. For each permuted dataset, let

$p^*_{(1)} \leq p^*_{(2)} \leq \cdots \leq p^*_{(K)}$ be the ordered unadjusted p-values. The adjusted p-value for the kth gene (not in the set whose adjusted p-values have already been set to zero) is then given by

$$\text{adjusted } p\text{-value}_k = \frac{1 + \# \text{ of random permutations where } p^*_{(U+1)} \leq p_k}{1 + \# \text{ of random permutations}}$$

or where it is possible to enumerate all permutations,

$$\text{adjusted } p\text{-value}_k = \frac{\# \text{ of permutations where } p^*_{(U+1)} \leq p_k}{\# \text{ of all possible permutations}}.$$

If one wants to be $100\,(1 - \alpha)$ percent confident that there are no more than U false positives, identify all genes with adjusted p-values $\leq \alpha$ (e.g., $\alpha = .05$). A schematic example of the method to identify differentially expressed genes to have 95% confidence that there are ≤ 10 false positives is given in Figure 7.5. Slight improvements on the procedure are possible using a stepwise modification; see Korn et al. (2003) for details. For the present application in which we expect that only a small percentage of a large number of genes is differentially expressed, this modification will have only a trivial effect on the adjusted p-values.

Example 7.8 (Genes showing differential expression in pre- and postchemotherapy gene expression in the Perou dataset: allowing for some false positives using a multivariate permutation approach). This is a continuation of Example 7.7. Allowing for at most two false positives with 95% confidence, the procedure identifies 28 genes.

7.3.3 Controlling the False Discovery Proportion

Rather than allowing for a certain number of false positives, suppose one wanted to control, out of those genes that are identified as being differentially expressed, the proportion that are false positives. We refer to this proportion as the *false discovery proportion*. For example, if 95 genes were identified as differentially expressed, of which 8 were false positives, then the false discovery proportion would be 0.084 ($= 8/95$). This subsection discusses two types of control of the false discovery proportion. First, we consider controlling the average of the false discovery proportion to be less than some value, for example, 0.10. (The average false discovery proportion is sometimes called the *false discovery rate*.) Secondly, we consider controlling the false discovery proportion to be less than some value with high confidence.

The methods described previously for controlling the number of false positives can be modified to control approximately the average false discovery proportion. Let $p_{(1)} \leq p_{(2)} \leq \cdots \leq p_{(K)}$ be the ordered unadjusted univariate p-values for the genes. To keep the average false discovery proportion less than γ, one identifies as differentially expressed those genes that are associated with

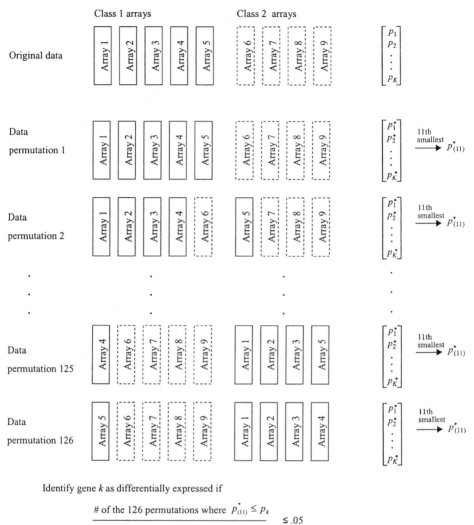

Identify gene k as differentially expressed if

$$\frac{\text{\# of the 126 permutations where } P^*_{(11)} \le p_k}{126} \le .05$$

Fig. 7.5. Schematic of method to identify differentially expressed genes for the two-class comparison (five observations in class 1 and four observations in class 2) in order to have 95% confidence that there are ≤ 10 false positives. The univariate p-values $p_1, \ldots, p_K$ correspond to two-sample t-statistics for the K genes on the microarray. (The ten genes with the smallest univariate p-values are also identified.)

indices $1, 2, \ldots, D$, where D is the largest index satisfying $(p_{(D)}K/D) < \gamma$. This procedure, based on the Bonferroni approach, has been studied by Benjamini and Hochberg (1995). (Note that D is the number of identified genes and $p_{(D)}K$ is an upper bound for the average number of false positives one would expect to see if one identified all genes with p-values less than $p_{(D)}$.)

Rather than using $p_{(D)}K$ as the estimator of the average number of false positives when estimating the average false discovery proportion, one could use the following procedure suggested by the work of Tusher et al. (2001). Consider any specific continuous measure of how differentially expressed a gene is, for example, the unadjusted univariate p-value. For a given cutoff on the measure, one can identify all genes that satisfy the cut-off, for example, all genes with unadjusted univariate p-values less than 0.001. One can estimate the average number of false positives using the same cutoff by permuting the specimen labels as previously described and averaging the number of identified genes over the different permutations. For a given cutoff, the average false discovery proportion is then estimated as the estimated average number of false positives divided by the number of genes identified on the original (unpermuted) data. One would then choose a cut-off yielding an acceptable average false discovery proportion, and identify all genes satisfying that cut-off. The SAM method uses this procedure with a measure of differential gene expression that uses a standardized mean difference in gene expression; see Tusher et al. (2001) for details.

Example 7.9 (Genes showing differential expression in pre- and postchemotherapy gene expression in the Perou dataset: controlling the false discovery proportion). This is a continuation of Example 7-8. With 8029 genes analyzed, allowing the average false discovery proportion to be 10%, 59 can be identified using the procedure studied by Benjamini and Hochberg (1995). The 59th smallest p-value is 0.00072 and $(8029 \times 0.00072)/59 = 0.098 < 10\%$, and this is the largest p-value that has this property.

In order to keep the false discovery proportion less than γ with a certain confidence, consider the genes in order from their smallest to largest p-value, that is, gene (k) is the one associated with $p_{(k)}$. For $|[k\gamma]| > |[(k-1)\gamma]|$, set the adjusted significance level of gene (k) to be 0, where the notation $|[x]|$ denotes the greatest integer less than or equal to x. For other values of k, using the permutations of the specimen labels as previously described, let

$$\text{adjusted } p\text{-value}_{(k)} = \frac{1 + \# \text{ of random permutations where } p^*_{(|[k\gamma]|+1)} \leq p_{(k)}}{1 + \# \text{ of random permutations}}$$

or where it is possible to enumerate all permutations,

$$\text{adjusted } p\text{-value}_{(k)} = \frac{\# \text{ of permutations where } p^*_{(|[k\gamma]|+1)} \leq p_k}{\# \text{ of all possible permutations}}.$$

To be $100(1-\alpha)\%$ confident that the false discovery proportion is no more than γ, identify all genes with adjusted p-values $\leq \alpha$. This procedure, and slight modifications of it, has been studied by Korn et al. (2003).

Example 7.10 (Genes showing differential expression in pre- and postchemotherapy gene expression in the Perou dataset: controlling the false discovery proportion using a multivariate permutation approach.). This is a continuation of Example 7.9. Constraining the false discovery proportion to be less than 10% with 95% confidence, we identify 28 genes as differentially expressed, which are the same 28 genes we identified in Example 7.8 when we allowed two false positives.

Whether to control for the number of false positives or to bound the false discovery proportion depends upon the investigation. For example, if one is willing to contend with up to 10 false positives in order to identify even only one or two truly differentially expressed genes, then controlling the number of false positives to be ≤ 10 is appropriate. On the other hand, if one desires to have a high proportion of the identified genes to be truly differentially expressed, then one should bound the false discovery proportion.

7.4 Experiments with Very Few Specimens from Each Class

As mentioned in Section 7.2, when there are few specimens available from each class the permutation t-tests will not be able to achieve small p-values and the parametric t-test may not be very efficient at identifying true class differences. An approach to this problem is to borrow strength from the data from other genes when examining class differences for a particular gene. One possible model that does this is

$$x_{ijk} = \lambda_i + \beta_k + \gamma_{ik} + e_{ijk} \qquad i = 1, \ldots, I \quad j = 1, \ldots, J_i \quad k = 1, \ldots, K, \quad (7.8)$$

where x_{ijk} is the (log-transformed) gene expression value for gene k for specimen j of class i. (We have in mind here two to five specimens per class. The special case of one specimen per class is qualitatively different and discussed in Section 7.6.) The parameters λ_i represent the overall effect of class i, and would be estimated to be close to zero if a normalization procedure were used that caused the average gene expression value to be about zero for each array (see Chapter 6). The parameters β_k are overall gene effects, representing that some genes are expressed more than others regardless of class. The interaction terms γ_{ik} are the ones of primary interest and represent class differences for the genes. They are constrained to sum to zero for each k, so that, for example, $\gamma_{1k} + \gamma_{2k} = 0$ with $I = 2$ classes. The error terms are assumed to have mean zero and to be independent of each other, and to have some additional distributional constraints. It is these additional constraints that allow one to pool information across the genes. For example, one might assume that the error terms are normally distributed with the same variance across all genes and specimens, or across all genes for specimens within a class. (The methods described below relax this assumption.) With this type of assumption, rather than estimating the variability for a given gene only from the small number of observations for that gene from the different specimens, thousands of observations (from all the genes) are used. The within-class variance is estimated separately for each gene, and then these gene-specific estimators are pooled. Analysis using model (7.8) then proceeds by estimating the interaction terms for each of the genes and obtaining a univariate p-value for each gene that it is differentially expressed. Because the analysis depends on the normality assumption, control for no false positives is problematic as described previously because the required accurate estimation of extremely small p-values will depend on the normality assumption holding perfectly. One can control for the average number of false positives as previously described, for example, by identifying all genes with univariate p-values < 0.001, or control for the average false discovery proportion. A more serious problem is the assumption that all genes have the same within-class variance of the log expression level. Although this may be a reasonable assumption for an analysis involving samples from a cell line in which the variability is mostly due to assay experimental error, it would not be a reasonable assumption for an analysis involving specimens from different patients in which the variability is mostly due to biological differences.

A different approach to borrowing strength involves *Bayesian methods* which relax the assumption that the variances of the genes are equal. Bayesian methods require specification of *prior distributions* for the model parameters. For example, one might assume that the log expression for a given gene and class are normally distributed with unknown mean and variance parameters. Then one specifies that these mean parameters come from a specified prior distribution and that the variance parameters come from a different specified prior distribution. In the implementation given in Baldi and Long (2001) for the two-class case, a very broad noninformative prior distribution is used for the mean parameters. The Baldi and Long approach yields univariate statistics for each gene that look like t-statistics except that the within-class variability is estimated as a weighted combination of the within-class variability of the gene under consideration and an estimate of the within-class variability from genes with expression levels similar to the gene under consideration; see Baldi and Long (2001) for details. A Bayesian approach is also described by Broet et al. (2002).

To avoid the requirement of specifying distributions on the parameters, Efron et al. (2001) use an *empirical Bayes* approach (for the two-class case). First, univariate statistics for each gene are calculated. These statistics look like t-statistics except that the within-class standard deviation is estimated as a weighted combination of the within-class standard deviation of the gene under consideration and the 90th percentile of the within-class standard deviations from all the other genes. The value of this statistic for each gene is then assumed to be a random selection from a mixture of two distributions: one for genes that are differentially expressed, and one from genes that are not differentially expressed; see also Lee et al. (2000). Rather than specifying these two distributions, the empirical distribution across the genes is used as an estimate of the mixture distribution, and the permutation distribution of statistics for comparing specimens within classes is used as an estimate of the distribution for genes that are not differentially expressed. The end result is an estimate for each gene of the probability that it is differentially expressed; see Efron et al. (2001) for details.

Wright and Simon (2003) developed a frequentist method for borrowing strength across the genes without assuming that all genes have the same within-class variance. They assume that the within-class variances for different genes are random draws for the same distribution. They use the entire dataset to estimate the parameters of this distribution. For the comparison of two classes, they derive a statistic that is very similar to the usual t-statistic except that the denominator contains an estimate of the standard error of the difference in class means based on a weighted average of the usual gene-specific variance estimate and an estimate based on the overall distribution average variance. They show that this statistic has a t-distribution, but with more degrees of freedom than the usual t-statistic based solely on the gene-specific variance. They also generalize this approach to the comparison of more than two classes and for analyzing the regression models described in Section 7.7.

Whatever statistical method is used to accommodate small numbers of specimens from each class, the ability to detect differentially expressed genes will be quite limited unless the within-class variability of gene expression is very small. Thus an analysis of a small number of arrays performed on samples of a cell line before and after an intervention may be informative about the effect of the intervention on gene expression because of the limited variability of gene expression expected from samples of a cell line. On the other hand, microarrays performed on a small number of breast cancers from patients who relapse early and from patients who remain relapse-free would be less likely to elucidate much about differences in gene expression between those two groups because of large expected variability in gene expression among breast cancers; see Section 7.6 for further discussion.

7.5 Global Tests of Gene Expression Differences Between Classes

In Section 7.3, we examined which genes among many were differentially expressed between classes. In this section we address a less ambitious question: Are the average gene expression levels different between the classes? Obviously, if one identified genes that were differentially expressed using the methods of Section 7.3, then one would have an affirmative answer to this question. But it is possible that one might be able to be confident that there are expression differences between the classes even though one could not be confident about which particular genes are differentially expressed. This could happen, for example, if no genes were strongly differentially expressed but many were modestly differentially expressed. In classical statistical applications where there are many more observations than variables, this type of global assessment of class differences would be addressed with a Hotelling's T^2-test (Johnson and Wichern 1999). This test, which has some optimality properties, requires calculating the inverses of the covariance matrix of the variables within each of the classes. In the present situation where each gene is a variable, there are thousands more variables than observations (specimens) and so Hotelling's T^2-test cannot be used. We instead consider some other statistics and a permutation-based approach to calculating the p-value for a global test.

Let T be a statistic calculated on the data from all the genes which has the property that its value increases as the difference between the classes becomes more pronounced. For example, T might be the sum over all the genes of some measure of differential gene expression (Chung and Fraser 1958) such as the square of the difference in class means divided by the pooled within-class variance estimator for that gene. Alternatively, T can be some other statistic that reflects class differences, for example, the number of genes that have unadjusted univariate p-values less than 0.01 based on a t-statistic. The statistic T is calculated on the original data as well as on datasets from random permutations of the specimen labels. Denoting the statistics calculated on the permuted datasets as T^*, the p-value is then given by

$$p\text{-value} = \frac{1 + \#\text{ of random permutations where } T^* \geq T}{1 + \#\text{ of random permutations}}$$

or where it is possible to enumerate all permutations,

$$p\text{-value} = \frac{\#\text{ of permutations where } T^* \geq T}{\#\text{ of all possible permutations}}.$$

As with the other permutation tests described previously in this chapter, the method of permutation of the specimen labels depends on the structure of the experiment. For example, with an (unpaired) two-class comparison with J_1 specimens in one class and J_2 specimens in the other, there are $\binom{J_1+J_2}{J_1}$ allowable permutations, whereas for a paired two-class comparison with J pairs of specimens, there are 2^J allowable permutations. Although the choice of T is up to the investigator, it has to be chosen before it is calculated on the data in order for the p-value to be valid. In other words, one cannot try a dozen different Ts and choose the one to report that yields the smallest p-value.

As mentioned at the beginning of this section, the reason for considering global tests of class differences is that they might have a greater ability to find class differences than the methods described in Section 7.3 which identify individual genes that distinguish the classes. However, investigators will rarely be satisfied solely with a global assessment that there are differences between classes but will want to know which genes are differentially expressed. In addition, frequently there are certain genes that are known a priori to be differentially expressed between the classes, so that a global assessment that classes differ in expression is not informative. These considerations suggest that applications in which global assessment will be useful are limited. One possible application would be to apply a global assessment to the genes remaining after those identified as being differentially expressed (using the techniques of Section 7.3) were removed from consideration. A positive global assessment would then suggest that additional studies with larger sample sizes might identify additional genes that were differentially expressed. Another possible application would be when one is focusing on a set of genes involved in a particular pathway. There may be interest in this situation in a global assessment of class differences in this set of genes.

7.6 Experiments with a Single Specimen from Each Class

Up to this point in this chapter, we have assumed that multiple specimens are available from each class for microarray analysis. These multiple specimens allow one to estimate the null hypothesis variability in mean differences (e.g., by permutation distributions) and thereby obtain p-values as described in the previous sections. In this section we review some methods that have been proposed for comparing expression profiles when there is only one specimen from each class. The valid information that can be obtained from such analyses is, however, generally very limited for the reasons described in Section 3.3. These methods all have the defect of supporting only a very narrow inference. That is, the conclusions only apply to the two RNA samples being compared. There is no way of estimating biological variability with only a single specimen per class and the results may even reflect differences in specimen handling and RNA extraction rather than biological effects.

Consider single microarrays done on a cell line before and after a manipulation. (With cDNA microarrays, there is the possibility of using one array with the test and reference samples corresponding to mRNA extractions from the cell line before and after the manipulation, respectively.) A naive approach would be to identify genes with a large difference in expression as being differentially expressed. But how large is large? Is a threefold difference large enough to be meaningful? Picking a fold cutoff too small will result in many genes being falsely identified as differentially expressed, especially considering the multiple comparisons involved.

Another unsatisfactory answer would be to identify the 5% of the genes with the largest differences; this would guarantee 5% of the total number of genes examined being falsely declared differentially expressed when there are actually no differences. If there is a set of predetermined housekeeping genes on the array that are not expected to be affected by the manipulation, then there is the possibility of using their values as a reference distribution (Chen et al. 1997; Chen 2002). In its simplest implementation, the difference in log-transformed expression values between the experimental conditions is calculated for each gene. Using this set of differences and normality assumptions, genes are identified as differentially expressed. This approach depends critically upon the normality assumption and the assumption that the housekeeping genes have the same background variability as all of the genes of interest.

Newton et al. (2001) suggest modeling the expression ratios from a single cDNA array. A parametric distribution is assumed for the joint density of the red and green intensities which are assumed to be statistically independent of each other as well as across spots. The intensities from an array are used to estimate the unknown parameters, which can then be used to estimate the ratio for any given spot in an empirical Bayes manner. This approach depends upon the assumption that red and green intensities are independent, which may be unrealistic.

If there are multiple spots for each gene on the microarrays then there are additional possible approaches, but they also are problematic. One approach is to treat the expression levels for the multiple spots as if they had come from different microarrays and then use the methods described previously in this chapter. To the extent that the array normalization is successful and provided that the multiple spots are not in one small area of the array, this is doable. (Multiple spots of the same gene on an array may be useful for other purposes such as quality control; see Section 5.3.2.)

With Affymetrix microarrays, there is the possibility of using the multiple probe pairs for each gene to examine specimen differences for that gene. For a single array from each of two specimens, the Affymetrix software calculates a p-value for each gene based on a Wilcoxon signed-rank test using the probe-pair-specific class differences between the perfect match and mismatch intensities, as well as the differences between the perfect match and background intensities; see Affymetrix (2001a) for details. Although the software uses these p-values to produce change calls, they should not be interpreted as p-values associated with hypothesis tests because there is no reason to assume that the probe-pair differences are statistically independent of each other (a requirement for the Wilcoxon signed-rank test to yield valid p-values). Instead, the p-values can be viewed as another way to rank the genes in terms of their differential expression between the specimens, or, stated more precisely, the differential expression between the two RNA extractions.

7.7 Regression Model Analysis; Generalizations of Class Comparison

The methods discussed up to this point in this chapter are for comparing gene expression between two or more classes. This goal is equivalent to examining the association of gene expression with a categorical variable representing the class membership of the specimen. A generalization of class comparison using regression models examines whether gene expression is associated with a continuous variable and/or multiple variables.

To define the models, it is convenient to change notation from that used previously in this chapter. For a single gene, let y_j be the (log-transformed) gene expression measurement for specimen j, $j = 1, 2, \ldots, J$. Gene expression would usually refer to either the normalized log signal for the Affymetrix array or the normalized log ratio for the two-color array in which the expression relative to a common, consistently labeled reference is used. We assume that the genes are being analyzed one at a time and do not use a subscript for the gene as this simplifies notation. A regression model corresponding to the two-class comparison discussed in previous sections of this chapter is

$$y_j = \alpha + \beta z_j + e_j, \tag{7.9}$$

where z_j is a binary $(0, 1)$ variable that is 0 if the jth specimen is in one class and 1 if it is in the other, and e_j is an error term. The *regression coefficient β* represents the average difference in gene expression between the classes. More generally, then *independent variable z_j* in model (7.9) could be a continuous variable corresponding to a phenotypic characteristic of specimen j. For example, z_j might be the systolic blood pressure of the individual from whom specimen j was obtained. With a continuous z_j, the coefficient β represents the average change in gene expression associated with a one-unit change in z_j. The null hypothesis that $\beta = 0$ represents no association between gene expression and the variable z. Assuming that the distribution of error terms is approximately normal or that the sample size is large, standard parametric methods can be used to estimate β and to calculate a test statistic and p-value associated with the null hypothesis (Draper and Smith 1998). Regardless of whether the error terms are approximately normally distributed or the sample size is large, a modification of the permutation methods described in Section 7.2 can be used to obtain a permutation p-value. Rather than permuting the class labels of the specimens, one permutes the values of the z among the specimens. That is, with J specimens, there are $J!$ permutations. When considering many genes, the regression model can be applied to each of the genes separately, and then the methods described in Section 7.3 (with $J!$ possible permutations) can be used to identify which genes are significantly associated with the variable z.

The model (7.9) can be further generalized to incorporate several phenotypic characteristics of the specimen or of the patient contributing the specimens. For example, the model could be

$$y_j = \alpha + \beta_1 z_j + \beta_2 w_j + e_j, \tag{7.10}$$

where z_j is the first phenotype characteristic for specimen j, and w_j is the second. Now there are two regression coefficients β_1 and β_2, one regression coefficient for each phenotypic characteristic. In this multivariate model, the value of β_1 represents the association between phenotype 1 and the gene expression for fixed values of the other phenotypic variable. This type of model is useful for exploring the relation of gene expression to a variable while controlling for the effect of a confounding variable that also affects gene expression. For example, if z_j is the cholesterol level and w_j is the body-mass-index of the individual from whom the jth specimen was obtained, then β_1 in (7.10) measures the association of gene expression and cholesterol level controlling for differences in body-mass-index. As another example, one may want to know whether gene expression is influenced by the presence of a BRCA1 mutation (z_j) if one controls for the effect of estrogen receptor status (w_j). Because BRCA1 status is correlated with estrogen receptor (ER) status and gene expression is associated with ER status, this type of multivariate regression may be useful for determining whether the association between gene expression and BRCA1 is independent of the effect of ER status.

Multivariate regression models such as (7.10) can also be useful for investigating the association of two phenotypes with gene expression even if those phenotypes are not correlated with each other. If phenotype 2 is strongly associated with gene expression, the multivariate regression model can be more effective in studying the association of phenotype 1 and gene expression than just a univariate analysis that ignores the effect of phenotype 2.

Multivariate regression models can incorporate more than two phenotypic characteristics, by having more than two independent variables on the right side of (7.10). However, as a rule of thumb, the total number of independent variables should be less than the sample size divided by 10 or 20 (Harrell 2001, p. 61).

7.8 Evaluating Associations of Gene Expression to Survival

In some studies it is important to identify the genes associated with survival. This type of data is frequently acquired in clinical trials or long-term observational studies, in which some observed individuals have not experienced the event (e.g., death) at the time of the analysis (i.e., are censored). Regression-type models, for example, the *proportional hazards regression model*, can be used to measure the association between the independent variables and the dependent variable survival. (Strictly speaking, the dependent "variable" is the *hazard* of experiencing the event at various timepoints. The hazard at any timepoint is the instantaneous rate of experiencing the event right after that time point given that the event has not occurred up until that timepoint. This hazard is what is modeled as a function of the independent variables.) The hazard function is not assumed constant over time. For the proportional hazards model, the logarithm of the ratio of hazards for any two individuals is assumed to be proportional to the independent variable. In the present context, the independent variable would be the gene expression. Standard statistical methods can be used to estimate the association and calculate a test statistic and p-value associated with the null hypothesis that the gene expression and survival times are unassociated (Marubini and Valsecchi 1995). A univariate proportional hazards model can be fit for evaluating the association of each gene to survival. Any of the multiple comparison methods described in Section 7.3 can be applied, using the p-values from the proportional hazards model. The permutation tests are based on permuting the survival times associated with the J expression profiles; again there are $J!$ possible permutations.

The proportional hazards regression model can be extended to include additional independent variables such as the stage of disease of the patients from whom the specimens were taken. The purpose of the analysis might be to identify genes that are predictive of survival independently of the standard disease staging system. The regression coefficients in these models (and more complex models) and p-values associated with these coefficients being zero can again be estimated by standard techniques (Marubini and Valsecchi 1995). When considering many genes, the models can be applied to one gene at a time. Some control for the multiple comparisons will usually be advisable to lessen the number of false discoveries, for example, selecting genes with unadjusted p-values $< .001$ as described in section 7.3. With multiple independent variables, however, it is not obvious how to adapt the permutation methods of Sections 7.2 and 7.3; this is an area of active research.

7.9 Models for Nonreference Designs on Dual-Label Arrays

Most of the analysis methods described in this chapter are applicable to either single-label arrays (eg., Affymetrix GeneChips^{TM}) or to dual-label arrays in which a common RNA reference specimen is consistently labeled with the same color label on each array (common reference design). Other designs, such as the loop and balanced block designs described in Chapter 3, are possible. As noted in Chapter 3, the balanced block design, illustrated in Figure 3.3, is sometimes very efficient for comparing two classes. Special methods are necessary for the analysis of such designs, however, because these designs involve the comparison of expression levels for specimens labeled with different dyes. With Affymetrix arrays, this obviously does not occur because only a single label is used. With two-color arrays utilizing the common reference design it also generally does not occur because all of the specimens of interest are labeled with the same color, the other color is used for the common reference. Although there may be some differential dye incorporation or differential dye detection effects not removed by normalization, they do not bias the comparison of classes using common reference designs because they affect all classes equally. This is not true of other types of designs for two-color arrays. Even for reference designs it is sometimes of secondary interest to compare gene expression in the experimental specimens to gene expression in the common reference. Such comparisons can be distorted by dye bias not removed by normalization and hence the methods presented in this section are useful for such comparisons.

In presenting methods for the comparison of classes with two-color arrays we have utilized the term "arrays" synonymously with "specimens" with the log ratio for a gene on an array being a measure of the expression of that gene in the experimental sample associated with the array. With designs that do not utilize common reference designs, this correspondence no longer exists and the analysis must be based on channel-specific intensities rather than log ratios. Models of this type have been studied by Kerr and Churchill (2001a), Wolfinger et al. (2001), Dobbin and Simon, (2002) and Dobbin et al. (2003). We utilize one of the models of Dobbin and Simon (2002) because it incorporates the effects of variability among specimens from individuals in the same class whereas many of the other models are designed to simply compare two RNA specimens or ignore the substantial variability among specimens from the same class. Dobbin et al. (2003) modeled background-subtracted channel-specific intensities. They applied this model after normalizing the intensities for each array. Their model is:

$$Y_{adcfg} = G_g + AG_{ag} + CG_{cg} + FG_{fg} + DG_{dg} + e_{adcfg}. \qquad (7.11)$$

Y_{adcfg} denotes the single-channel log intensity for gene g for a sample from individual f of class c, labeled with dye d, and hybridized on array a. Although we include the subscript g for gene, a model is fit separately for each gene.

The class-by-gene interactions CG_{cg} are the terms of interest. The array-by-gene interactions AG_{ag} are the "spot effects." These reflect the fact that the intensity of corresponding spots on two different arrays may differ because of differences in the sizes of the spots and the distribution of the samples on the two arrays. These spot effects influence both samples similarly. The main advantage of a common reference design is that these spot effects are eliminated by the calculation of the log ratios used to analyze such designs. The balanced block design and loop design discussed in Section 3.6 also control the spot effects. Spot effects can be quite large for cDNA arrays. Use of designs for cDNA arrays that require the spot effects to be incorporated in the error term is not recommended as it can substantially decrease the statistical power for detecting differences in gene expression among classes.

The sample-by-gene interactions FG_{fg} represent the variability among individuals of the same class with regard to expression of the gene. Without the FG_{fg} terms one would be ignoring the distinction between sampling of individuals and subsampling of RNA for a single individual. The dye-by-gene interactions DG_{dg} represent the gene-specific dye biases that may remain after normalization. Although such effects may exist for many genes, they are usually small. As discussed in Chapter 3, however, if there is interest in comparing experimental samples to a common reference, the comparison must be adjusted with regard to dye-by-gene interactions. The model (7.11) provides an approach to producing such adjusted estimates.

These models are analyzed separately for each gene on the array using standard analysis of variance or mixed model statistical software. The objective is to determine which genes show statistically significant gene-by-class interactions. In order to control for multiple comparisons, statistical significance at the $p < 0.001$ level should be required or some other multiple testing procedure implemented for controlling the number or percentage of false discoveries. Some investigators have suggested fitting one large analysis of variance model that combines all genes and to assume that the residual error terms have a variance that is the same for all genes, but in our experience this is not a good assumption. It is also computationally much simpler to fit the models separately for each gene.

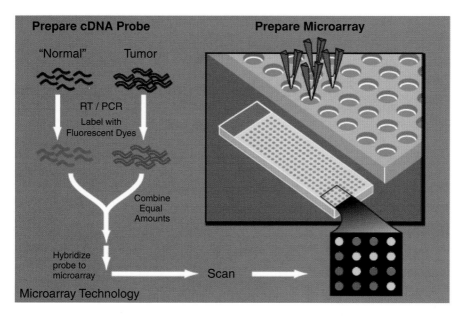

Plate 1 (Figure 2.1) Schematic of robotic printing of spots for cDNA array (right) and of processing of rna samples for co-hybridization to array.

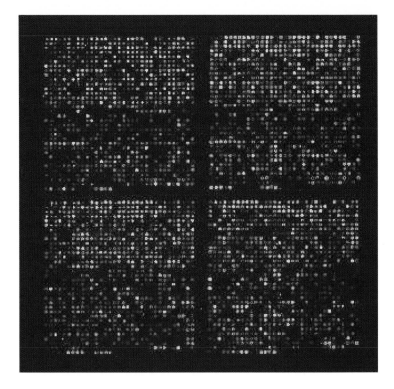

Plate 2 (Figure 2.2) A typical cDNA microarray image with two rows and two columns of grids.

Reference Design

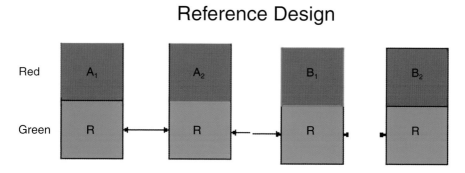

Plate 3 (Figure 3.2) Reference design. Aliquot of reference sample is labeled with the same label and used on each array.

Balanced Block Design

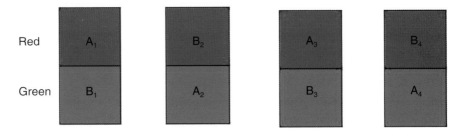

Plate 4 (Figure 3.3) Balanced block design for comparing two classes of samples. Each array contains a biologically independent sample from each class. Each class is labeled on half the arrays with one label and on the other half of the arrays with the other label. Each biologically independent sample is hybridized to a single array.

Loop Design

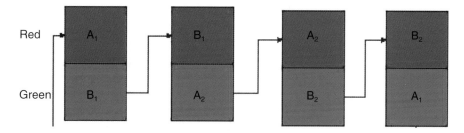

Plate 5 (Figure 3.4) Loop design for comparing two classes of samples. Each biologically independent sample is sub-aliquoted and hybridized to two arrays, once with the Cy3 label and once with the Cy5 label. Each array contains a sample from each class.

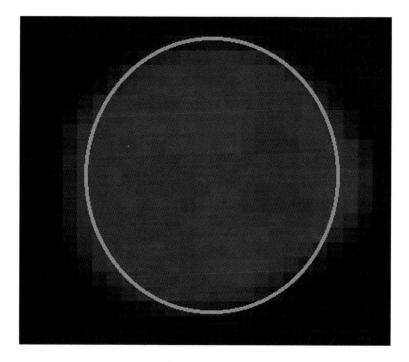

Plate 6 (Figure 4.1) An enlarged spot patch shown at pixel level. The spot is non-circular shaped, with a circular mask placed for segmentation.

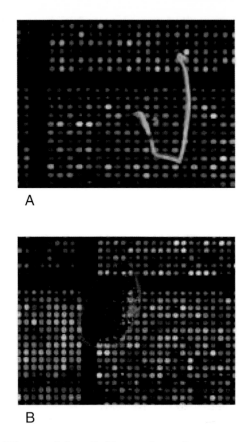

A

B

Plate 7 and 8 (Figure 5.1a–d) Examples of array anomalies that can be detected through examination of the Image file. a) Bright streak indicating the presence of a fiber on the array. b) Dark patch indicating the presence of a bubble on the array.

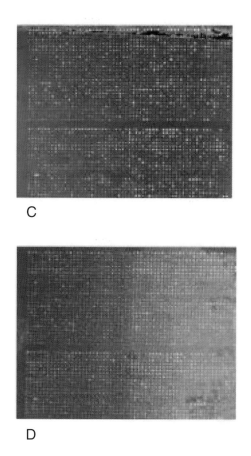

C

D

Plate 7 and 8 (Figure 5.1a–d) *continued*: c) Background subtraction may be able to correct for the uniform green haze covering slide, but spots covered by red haze along top should be excluded. d) Background subtraction alone may not be able to account for strong green haze on right side of slide. Location normalization is recommended.

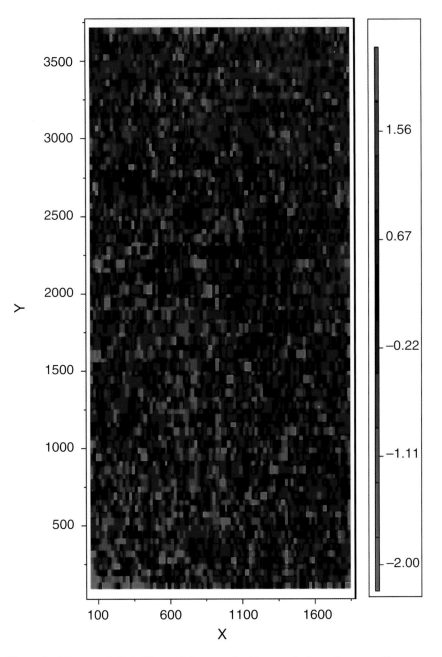

Plate 9 (Figure 6.2a) Plot of log-ratio for each location on the
array before normalization. High enrichment for red along the top
and right sides, indicate possible need for location based normalization.

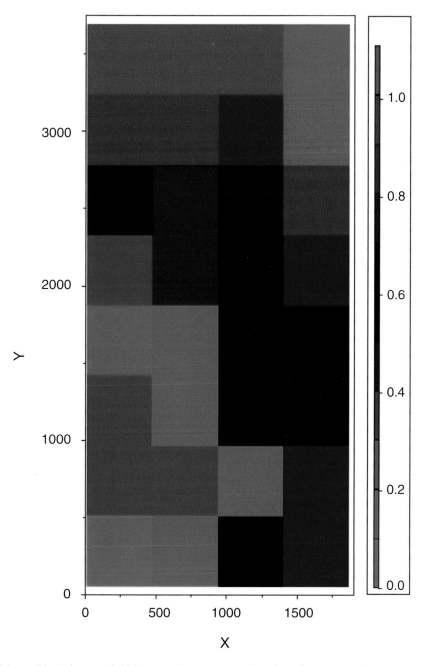

Plate 10 (Figure 6.2b) Location normalization factors of each grid for array depicted in figure 6.2a

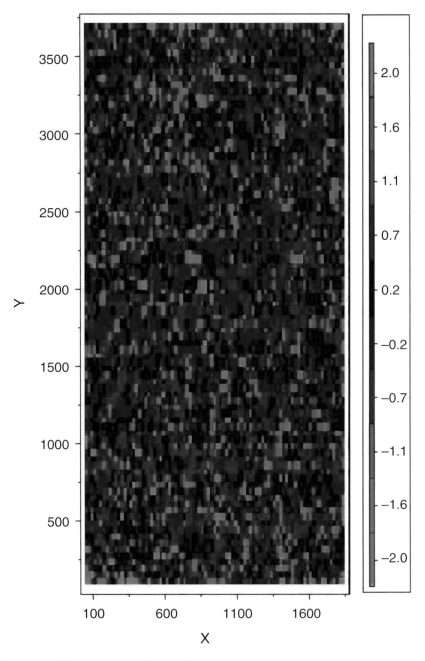

Plate 11 (Figure 6.2c) Plot of log-ratio for each location on the array after location based normalization. Red and green signals are now dispersed evenly across slide.

MDS: Breast Tumor and FNA Samples

Color = Patient
Large circle = Tumor
Small circle = FNA

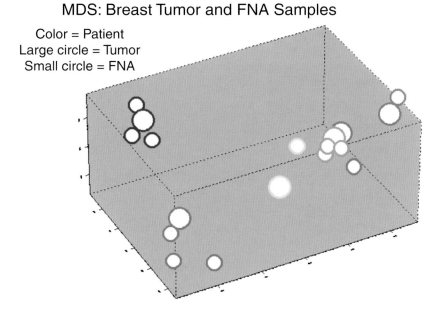

Plate 12 (Figure 9.4) Multidimensional scaling display of the gene expression profiles obtained for a collection of breast tumor specimens (large circles) and fine needle aspirate specimens (small circles). Data are from Assersohn et al., (2002). Different colors represent different patients. The distance metric used in the multidimensional scaling was one minus the Pearson correlation.

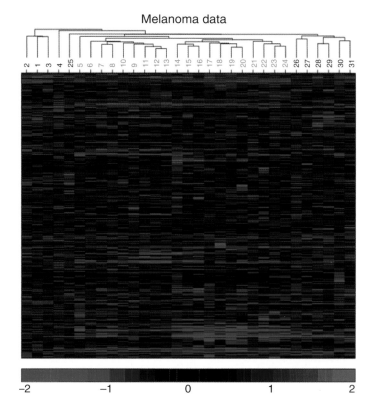

Plate 13 (Figure 9.8) Color image plot representing results of average linkage hierarchical cluster analysis of gene expression profiles obtained for 31 melanoma tumors (Bittner et al., 2000). Distance metric was one minus Pearson correlation. Tumors (columns) and genes (rows) are each ordered according to dendrogram order. At the top is the dendrogram resulting from the clustering of the tumors. Because the distance metric used for clustering was 1-correlation, each block in this display has been color-coded by the value of its corresponding standardized log ratio (for each log expression ratio on each array, subtract the mean log expression ratio for the array and divide by the standard deviation for the array). Blocks colored most intense red represent the most highly over-expressed genes, and blocks colored most intense green represent the genes with greatest degree of under-expression. Black indicates genes whose expression is similar in the experimental and common reference samples. Note the red band of blocks (corresponding to a subset of genes) at the center top of the image plot. This appears to be one of the defining characteristics of the subgroup of tumors consisting of tumors 5-24 with tumor numbers printed in orange.

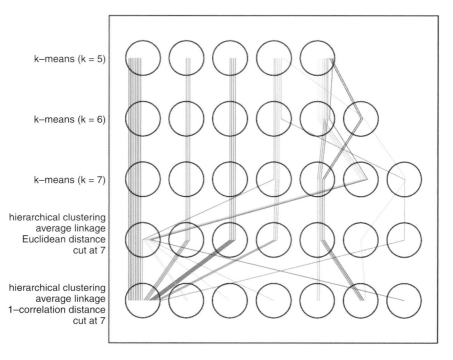

k—means (k = 5)

k—means (k = 6)

k—means (k = 7)

hierarchical clustering
average linkage
Euclidean distance
cut at 7

hierarchical clustering
average linkage
1—correlation distance
cut at 7

Plate 14 (Figure 9.9) Parallel coordinates plot displaying results of multiple clustering methods applied to the melanoma data of Bittner et al. (2000). The first (lowest) level of circles represents the clusters derived by hierarchical clustering using distance of one minus Pearson correlation and average linkage; the left-most cluster is the 20-element cluster of tumors 5-24 noted in Figure 9.3. The second level shows the clusters derived from hierarchical clustering with average linkage using Euclidean distance rather than one minus correlation distance. The third through fifth levels are based on k-means clustering with k = 7, 6, and 5, respectively. Each k-means result is the best obtained (smallest sum of squared distances from centroids) from among ten separate k-means analyses, each using a different set of k initial cluster centroids selected randomly from among the 31 tumor profiles.

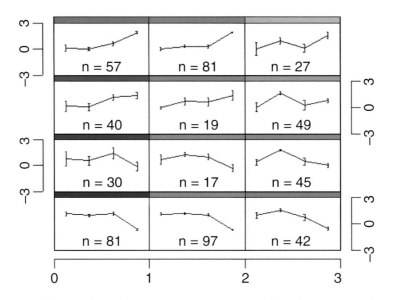

Plate 15 (Figure 9.10) Profile plots obtained for the nodes of a 4 by 3 SOM constructed to cluster genes in a time course experiment involving hematopoietic differentiation in HL-60 cells (Tamayo et al., 1999). Plotted values represent average log base 2 expression measurements, and error bars represent one standard deviation. The value of n designated for each node is the number of genes that were mapped to that node by the SOM analysis.

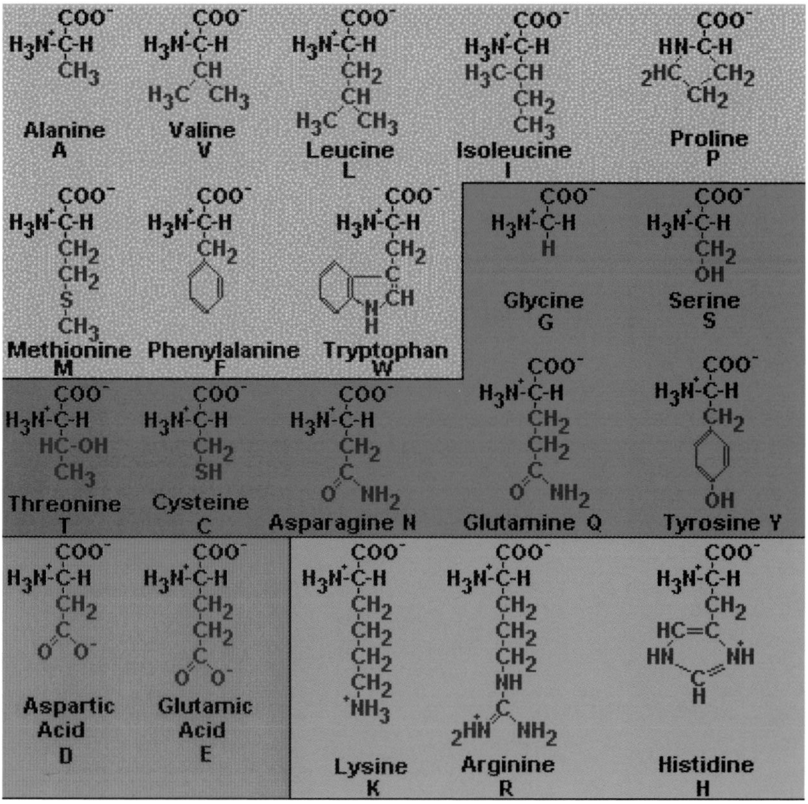

Plate 16 (Figure A.2).

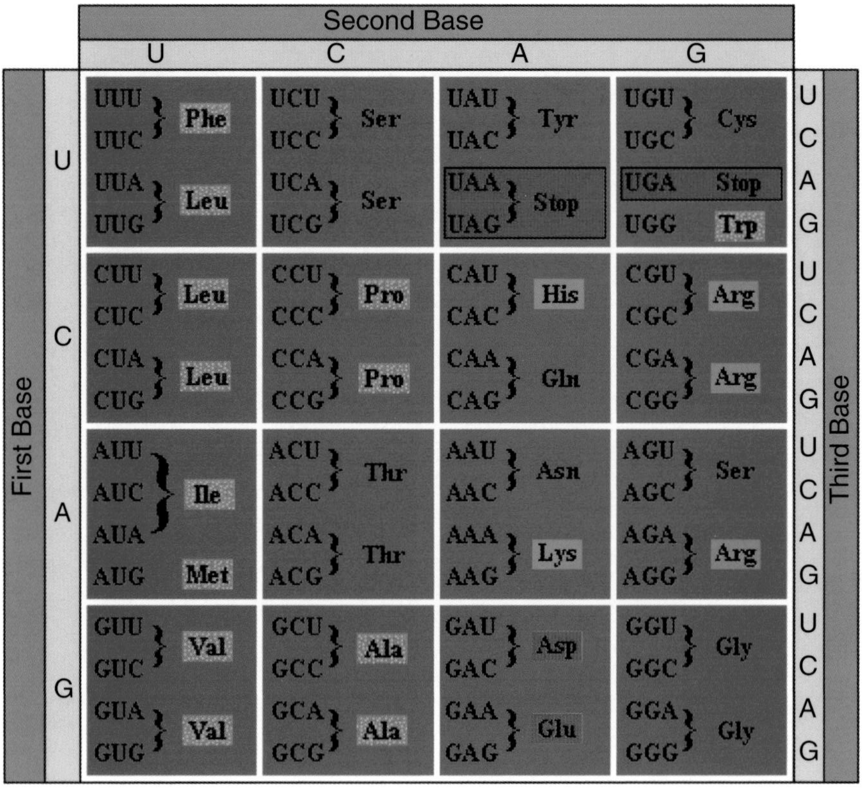

		Second Base				
		U	C	A	G	
First Base	U	UUU } Phe UUC UUA } Leu UUG	UCU } Ser UCC UCA } Ser UCG	UAU } Tyr UAC UAA } Stop UAG	UGU } Cys UGC UGA Stop UGG Trp	U C A G
	C	CUU } Leu CUC CUA } Leu CUG	CCU } Pro CCC CCA } Pro CCG	CAU } His CAC CAA } Gln CAG	CGU } Arg CGC CGA } Arg CGG	U C A G
	A	AUU AUC } Ile AUA AUG Met	ACU } Thr ACC ACA } Thr ACG	AAU } Asn AAC AAA } Lys AAG	AGU } Ser AGC AGA } Arg AGG	U C A G
	G	GUU } Val GUC GUA } Val GUG	GCU } Ala GCC GCA } Ala GCG	GAU } Asp GAC GAA } Glu GAG	GGU } Gly GGC GGA } Gly GGG	U C A G

(Right side label: Third Base)

Plate 17 (Figure A.5).

8

Class Prediction

8.1 Introduction

In this chapter, we address statistical methods for *class prediction* and *prognostic prediction* using microarray data. For class prediction, the goal is to develop a multivariate class predictor for accurately predicting class membership (phenotype) of a new individual (specimen). Similar to class comparison studies (Chapter 7), it is required that supplemental class information be available for each individual in the dataset from which the predictor will be built. For example, breast tissue specimens may be classified as either normal or cancer. In some cases, prognostic prediction is encompassed by class prediction. For example, to predict which patients will respond to a specified treatment we can consider two classes consisting of responders and nonresponders, respectively. There are other situations where prognostic prediction based on gene expression profiles is not encompassed by the class prediction paradigm. For example, in many cases outcome is measured by survival time or some other time-to-event measurement, and it is desired to develop a prognostic index based on gene expression measurements that will be related to that outcome. Such predictors can aid in many types of clinical management decisions such as risk assessment, diagnostic testing, prognostic stratification for clinical trials, and treatment selection. Sometimes prognostic prediction problems are converted to class prediction problems by creating prognostic classes defined by applying cutpoints to the outcome variable, for example, short-term (< 5 years) survivors versus long-term (> 5 years) survivors.

There is a large literature of methods for developing multivariate predictors of class membership. These methods include logistic regression (Cox 1970), linear and quadratic discriminant analysis (Johnson and Wichern 1999), nearest-neighbor classifiers (Hastie et al. 2001), decision trees (Breiman et al. 1984), neural networks (Ripley 1996), support-vector machines (Vapnik 1998), and many others. Unfortunately, none of these methods was developed in the context of studies in which the number of candidate predictors is at least one order of magnitude larger than the number of cases. Sophisticated methods that work well to uncover structure and provide accurate predictors when the number of cases is large relative to the number of candidate predictors often work very poorly in the opposite situation when the number of cases is small relative to the number of predictors. Furthermore, in this latter situation, if a predictor's accuracy is assessed by testing it on the same data from which it was derived, it will virtually always show excellent prediction accuracy, but it will perform poorly on new data. This phenomenon is known as *overfitting*, and it occurs because too many parameters are being fit to too few datapoints, resulting in fitting to random noise in the data. In Section 8.4 we discuss how to obtain more accurate estimates of predictor performance.

Some investigators have tried to justify the use of cluster analysis for class prediction as a way to avoid the overfitting problem because the class information plays no role in deriving the predictor. However, ignoring the class information that is available will often come at great expense to the performance of the predictor. Genes that distinguish classes may be few in number and their influence may be lost in a cluster analysis that is based on a distance metric utilizing information from the full set of analyzed genes.

In the following sections, we describe several class prediction methods and apply them to some microarray data examples. To simplify the discussion, we focus on the development of predictors for classifying specimens into one of two classes, for example, classifying breast tissue specimens as normal versus cancer. We suppose that for each of J specimens there is a K-dimensional vector of gene expression measurements and an indicator of class membership. Let $x_j = (x_{j1}, x_{j2}, \ldots, x_{jK})$ denote the K-gene expression profile for specimen j. For Affymetrix GeneChips^{TM} these expression measurements will usually be log signal values and for two-color arrays based on common reference designs they will usually be log ratios (see Section 3.6.1). Let y_j be the class label for specimen j. We assume that the expression data have already been appropriately filtered and normalized (Chapters 5 and 6). Following presentation of the various methods for building predictors in Sections 8.2 and 8.3, we discuss methods for obtaining accurate estimates of prediction accuracy and for assessing "statistical significance" of a predictor in Section 8.4. In Section 8.5 we compare the methods and give a worked example. Finally, we discuss the extension of class prediction methods to developing a gene expression-based prognostic index for predicting survival outcome in Section 8.6.

Some parts of Section 8.3 contain more mathematical notation than other sections of this book. This is done in order to show the similarities among several of the commonly used class prediction methods. This section should be understandable to the nonmathematical reader, however, even if the formulas are skipped.

8.2 Feature Selection

Feature selection is a common first step when developing a class predictor based on microarray data. It is a key step; often, selection of the important genes for inclusion in the model is more important than the specific way that their influence is modeled. Most effective predictive models require a feature selection step.

It is generally reasonable to assume that only some subset of the many measured genes contribute useful information for distinguishing the classes. One approach to feature selection, therefore, is to select genes based on their statistical significance in univariate tests of differences between the classes. For this purpose, t-tests or Wilcoxon rank-sum tests described in Chapter 7 can be used to assess univariate statistical significance. The most statistically significant genes are selected for inclusion in the multivariate model. Increasing the stringency of the significance threshold results in a simpler model containing fewer genes, but risks missing important genes. It may require larger sample sizes to identify the most important genes than to develop a model that accurately predicts based on inclusion of a larger number of genes. One strategy is to experiment with significance thresholds ranging from 0.01 to 0.0001 and determines the cross-validated misclassification rate (see Section 8.4.2) for the resulting models.

Missing data are a common occurrence in gene expression profiling studies and data imputation is sometimes necessary (see Chapter 5). For class prediction analyses, imputation should generally not be performed before feature selection. For example, imputation is unnecessary prior to a two-sample t-test for selecting differentially expressed genes. The t-statistic for a given gene can simply be computed based on the available data. Imputation prior to feature selection likely adds superfluous noise to the analysis and may even bias the estimate of prediction accuracy.

An alternative to selecting individual genes is to utilize the first several principal components (Section 9.3) of the genes (Khan et al. 2001; West et al. 2001). This would greatly reduce the number of predictors but the principal components are not necessarily good predictors of class membership. Partial least squares analysis is another method for identifying a small number of linear combinations of individual gene expression vectors for use in the predictive model (Nguyen et al. 2002). Partial least squares analysis selects linear combinations of the genes that maximize the covariance with the class label variable. These types of dimension reduction methods have disadvantages, however. For example, linear combinations of thousands of genes are difficult to interpret and using linear combinations as predictors does not reduce the number of genes that need to be measured in subsequent studies. Also, these methods cannot easily handle missing data, necessitating a data imputation step prior to feature selection (see Chapter 5).

8.3 Class Prediction Methods

Here we provide an overview of some of the many methods that have been used for class prediction using gene expression profiles. Many class prediction problems involve two groups or can be reduced to a two-group classification by combining similar groups or by performing a sequence of two-group classifications. Thus the methods are described in the context of two-group prediction.

8.3.1 Nomenclature

We assume each of J specimens in the training set has a gene expression profile containing expression intensity measurements for the G genes selected during the feature selection step. Let $\mathbf{x}_j = (x_{j1}, x_{j2}, \ldots, x_{jG})'$ represent the gene expression profile for specimen j, and let y_j be the class label for specimen j. (To simplify presentation of models, we assume that the feature variables correspond to individual genes, but in general, the feature values could be composites of gene values, for example, principal components or average expression values for gene clusters. The feature variables should not, however, be computed based on the class labels.) The class labels are either 1 or 2 depending on the class of the specimen. A parenthetical superscript denotes a class-specific parameter and a bar above a parameter denotes the arithmetic mean of the parameter. For example, the mean expression profile for training-set specimens with $y = 1$ is denoted by $\bar{\mathbf{x}}^{(1)}$.

8.3.2 Discriminant Analysis

The expression profile of a specimen may contain many genes even if the expression matrix is limited to contain only those genes that are individually differentially expressed between classes. Trying to define complex prediction regions in this high-dimensional space may require many specimens. An alternative is to create a function that summarizes the high-dimensional information on a one-dimensional scale and base prediction to one of the two classes on the summary measure. Discriminant analysis is a method for doing this (see Figure 8.1).

Fisher (1936) developed a method for the solution of the two-group classification problem known as linear discriminant analysis. In Fisher linear discriminant analysis, the gene expression profile $\mathbf{x}_j$ of a specimen is reduced to a single scalar value by computing a linear combination of its elements:

$$z_j = u_1 x_{j1} + u_2 x_{j2} + \cdots + u_K x_{jG}, \tag{8.1}$$

where the u values are the weights for the specific genes in the linear combination. The same weights are used for all specimens. The linear combination can be written in matrix notation as $z_j = \mathbf{u}'\mathbf{x}_j$, where $\mathbf{u}' = (u_1, u_2, \ldots, u_G)$. The objective of Fisher linear discriminant analysis is to find a set of weights

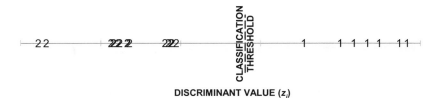

DISCRIMINANT VALUE (z_j)

Fig. 8.1. Discriminant analysis for prediction involving two classes. The multidimensional gene expression profile of each specimen is summarized by a linear combination of the individual expression measurements that compose the profile (weights are chosen for the linear combination such that maximal separation between the two classes is obtained). The summary measures (known as discriminant values) for specimens in class 1 or class 2 are indicated on the graph by a **1** or **2**, respectively. The classification threshold is based on the within-class distributions of the discriminant values (here the midpoint of the class means is used as in linear discriminant analysis). A new specimen is classified by computing its discriminant value and determining on what side of the threshold it falls (assigned to class 1 if greater than the threshold and to class 2 if less than the threshold).

(i.e., the elements of the weight vector $\mathbf{u}$) so that the linear combination of gene expressions maximally discriminates between profiles of the two classes in the training set.

The criterion for maximal discrimination, as Fisher defined it, is to find the linear combination that has the largest absolute difference in means between the two classes, relative to the within-class variability. Thus the target summary measure is one that possesses the largest difference, on average, between specimens of class 1 and class 2 when standardized by the natural variation in the summary measure. The value of $\mathbf{u}$ that satisfies this maximal discrimination criterion is

$$\mathbf{u}' = \mathbf{d}'\mathbf{S}^{-1}, \tag{8.2}$$

where $\mathbf{d} = \bar{\mathbf{x}}^{(1)} - \bar{\mathbf{x}}^{(2)}$ is a vector containing the average differences in expression of all selected genes between the two classes and $\mathbf{S}$ denotes the pooled within-class covariance matrix of the expression levels of the genes. A covariance matrix is a multivariate generalization of a variance. In fact, the diagonal elements of $\mathbf{S}$ are simply the pooled within-class sample variances of the genes. So the value of the summary measure (also known as the discriminant function) for specimen j is

$$z_j = \mathbf{d}'\mathbf{S}^{-1}\mathbf{x}_j. \tag{8.3}$$

Classification of a new specimen with expression profile $\mathbf{x}$ is a matter of computing the value of the discriminant function for the new specimen and determining to which class mean it is closer. The new specimen is assigned to class 1 if $z = \mathbf{d}'\mathbf{S}^{-1}\mathbf{x}$ is closer to $\mathbf{d}'\mathbf{S}^{-1}\bar{\mathbf{x}}^{(1)}$ than it is to $\mathbf{d}'\mathbf{S}^{-1}\bar{\mathbf{x}}^{(2)}$; otherwise, it is assigned to class 2. Equivalently, consider the statistic

$$W = \mathbf{d}'\mathbf{S}^{-1}\left(\mathbf{x} - \frac{1}{2}\left(\bar{\mathbf{x}}^{(1)} + \bar{\mathbf{x}}^{(2)}\right)\right) \tag{8.4}$$

and assign the new specimen to class 1 if $W > 0$ and to class 2 otherwise.

Fisher linear discriminant analysis is a nonparametric method: no distributional assumptions are made concerning the gene expression profiles of the two classes. In order to apply Fisher linear discriminant analysis, however, one must compute $\mathbf{S}$, the covariance matrix of the genes, and then invert it. This means that the number of genes G passing the feature selection stage must be less than the number of specimens available, or else the covariance matrix will not be invertible. Even if G is less than the number of specimens J, there are $G(G+1)/2$ variances and covariances to be estimated using the J specimens in addition to the G expression means in each class. Hence Fisher linear discriminant analysis requires estimation of a large number of parameters for microarray studies. If there are only 20 genes selected for inclusion in the model ($G = 20$), then there are 420 variances and covariances to estimate in addition to the 40 means.

Other forms of discriminant analysis exist and may be used for class prediction in place of Fisher linear discriminant analysis. Typically, the two classes of gene expression profiles are assumed to have distinct multivariate Gaussian densities with a mean vector $\boldsymbol{\mu}^{(1)}$ in class 1 and mean vector $\boldsymbol{\mu}^{(2)}$ in class 2. Similarly, there is a covariance matrix $\Sigma^{(1)}$ for class 1 and a covariance matrix $\Sigma^{(2)}$ for class 2. For each class, the mean vector and covariance matrix must be estimated from the training set: the sample estimates $\bar{\mathbf{x}}^{(k)}$ and $\mathbf{S}^{(k)}$ are used in place of $\boldsymbol{\mu}^{(k)}$ and $\Sigma^{(k)}$, respectively. Using the parameter estimates, the multivariate Gaussian probability density of the observation to be classified is computed for each class. The specimen is classified into that class for which the probability density is largest. The data in the training set are utilized only for computing the estimates of the class-specific mean vectors and covariance matrices. This method is known as quadratic discriminant analysis (Johnson and Wichern, 1999). If the covariance matrices in the two classes are assumed to be equal, then the method is equivalent to Fisher linear discriminant analysis.

Two other special cases of discriminant analysis are worthy of attention; both assume that class densities have diagonal covariance matrices (i.e., each pair of genes has correlation equal to zero). Although the assumption of diagonal covariance matrices is surely biologically incorrect (gene networks and coregulation are well-established principles of genetics), the assumption leads to simplified analyses and, as discussed in Section 8.3.7, may result in better prediction accuracy than standard discriminant rules. In one case, the two classes have distinct covariance matrices and the method is known as *diagonal quadratic discriminant analysis*. In the other case, known as *diagonal linear discriminant analysis*, not only are gene covariances assumed to be zero, the variances are assumed to be the same for the two classes. The new sample, represented by a vector $\mathbf{x}$ of expression measurements, is assigned to class 1 if

$$\sum_{i=1}^{G} \left[\frac{\left(x_i - \bar{x}_i^{(1)}\right)^2}{s_i^2} \right] \leq \sum_{i=1}^{G} \left[\frac{\left(x_i - \bar{x}_i^{(2)}\right)^2}{s_i^2} \right] \qquad (8.5)$$

and otherwise it is assigned to class 2. In this formula, s_i^2 denotes the pooled estimate of the within-class variance for gene i, $\bar{x}_i^{(1)}$ and $\bar{x}_i^{(2)}$ denote the mean expression of gene i in classes 1 and 2, respectively, and x_i denotes the expression for gene i in the sample to be classified. This diagonal linear discriminant rule can be based on the statistic W as was done for Fisher linear discriminant analysis in Equation (8.4). For diagonal linear discrimination,

$$W = \mathbf{d}'\mathbf{S}^{-1} \left(\mathbf{x} - \frac{1}{2}\left(\bar{\mathbf{x}}^{(1)} + \bar{\mathbf{x}}^{(2)}\right) \right)$$

$$= \sum_{i=1}^{G} \frac{\left(\bar{x}_i^{(1)} - \bar{x}_i^{(2)}\right)}{s_i^2} \left(x_i - \frac{1}{2}\left(\bar{x}_i^{(1)} + \bar{x}_i^{(2)}\right) \right) \qquad (8.6)$$

and the specimen is assigned to class 1 if $W > 0$ and to class 2 otherwise. Diagonal linear discriminant analysis requires only the estimation of G variances in addition to the $2G$ means. Hence for $G = 20$, only 20 variances must be estimated instead of 420 elements of the covariance matrix as in Fisher's linear discriminant analysis.

8.3.3 Variants of Diagonal Linear Discriminant Analysis

8.3.3.1 Golub's Weighted Vote Method

Golub et al. (1999) developed a prediction method in which a fixed number n_s of genes informative in the two-class distinction in a training set cast weighted votes for classification of new specimens. Informative genes are defined as those most highly correlated with the class distinction, where the correlation of gene j with the class label is defined by

$$P_j = \frac{\bar{x}_j^{(1)} - \bar{x}_j^{(2)}}{s_j^{(1)} + s_j^{(2)}}. \qquad (8.7)$$

P_j is similar in form to the two-sample t-statistic (though the denominator of P_j is not an appropriate form for the standard error of the mean difference). An equal number of genes with high expression in class 1 relative to class 2 and low expression in class 1 relative to class 2 comprise the informative gene set. This is accomplished by including the $n_s/2$ genes with largest values of P_j and the $n_s/2$ genes with largest values of $-P_j$ in the informative gene set. Each of the genes then casts a "weighted vote" for class prediction, with the weighted vote of gene i equal to

$$v_i = P_i\left(x_i - \frac{1}{2}\left(\bar{x}_i^{(1)} + \bar{x}_i^{(2)}\right)\right)$$

$$= \frac{\left(\bar{x}_i^{(1)} - \bar{x}_i^{(2)}\right)}{s_i^{(1)} + s_i^{(2)}}\left(x_i - \frac{1}{2}\left(\bar{x}_i^{(1)} + \bar{x}_i^{(2)}\right)\right), \tag{8.8}$$

where a positive value of v_i indicates a vote for class 1 and a negative value indicates a vote for class 2. The sum of all votes is

$$V = \sum_{i=1}^{n_s} \frac{\bar{x}_i^{(1)} - \bar{x}_i^{(2)}}{s_i^{(1)} + s_i^{(2)}}\left(x_i - \frac{1}{2}\left(\bar{x}_i^{(1)} + \bar{x}_i^{(2)}\right)\right) \tag{8.9}$$

with prediction to class 1 when $V > 0$ and to class 2 otherwise. Comparison to Equation (8.6) indicates that Golub's weighted vote method is a variant of the diagonal linear discriminant rule, with the sample pooled variance s_i^2 (the denominator in the sum) replaced by the sum of the two within-class standard errors $s_i^{(1)} + s_i^{(2)}$.

8.3.3.2 Compound Covariate Predictor

Tukey (1993) proposed the use of compound covariates in clinical trials for which for which there may be several dozen covariates and a few hundred patients. A compound covariate is a linear combination of the basic covariates being studied, with each covariate having its own coefficient or weight in the linear combination. The microarray setting is far more extreme than what Tukey envisioned, typically thousands of covariates and a few to several dozen patients. Nonetheless, the compound covariate method has proven to be useful for class prediction using microarray data when applied to genes differentially expressed in the two-class comparison (Hedenfalk et al.2001; Radmacher et al. 2002).

Selection of differentially expressed genes is based on a two-sample t-test of gene expression measurements for the two classes of specimens in the training set. Either a predetermined number of genes with largest t-statistics (in absolute value) form the set of differentially expressed genes, or a variable number of genes significant in the t-test at a predetermined significance level form the set. With the differentially expressed genes determined, a single compound covariate is formed with the two-sample t-statistic of each differentially expressed gene serving as its weight in the compound covariate. Thus the value of the compound covariate for specimen j is

$$c_j = \sum_{i=1}^{G} t_i x_{ji}, \tag{8.10}$$

where t_i is the t-statistic for the two group comparison with respect to gene i, x_{ji} is the log expression measurement in specimen j for gene i, and the sum is over all selected genes.

Once the value of the compound covariate is computed for each specimen in the training set, a classification threshold C_t is calculated:

$$C_t = \frac{\bar{c}^{(1)} + \bar{c}^{(2)}}{2},$$

(8.11)

where $\bar{c}^{(1)}$ and $\bar{c}^{(2)}$ are the mean values of the compound covariate for specimens of class 1 and class 2 in the training set, respectively. In other words, C_t is the midpoint of the means of the two classes. A new specimen is predicted to be of class 1 if its compound covariate is closer to $\bar{c}^{(1)}$ and to be of class 2 if its value is closer to $\bar{c}^{(2)}$.

When there are no missing data, compound covariate prediction can be performed based on the statistic

$$C = \sum_i \frac{\bar{x}_i^{(1)} - \bar{x}_i^{(2)}}{s_i} \left(x_i - \frac{1}{2} \left(\bar{x}_i^{(1)} + \bar{x}_i^{(2)} \right) \right),$$

(8.12)

where $(\bar{x}_i^{(1)} - \bar{x}_i^{(2)})/s_i$ is the form of the two-sample t-statistic (ignoring a factor in the denominator related to sample size that is constant with respect to i and, hence, does not affect prediction). Prediction is to class 1 if $C > 0$ and class 2 otherwise. Comparison of Equation (8.12) to Equation (8.6) indicates that compound covariate prediction is another variant of diagonal linear discriminant analysis with the sample pooled variance s_i^2 (the denominator in Equation (8.6)) replaced by its square root s_i. The difference in W and C indicates that diagonal linear discriminant analysis gives higher weight to genes with smaller within-class variance estimates given the same fold difference.

8.3.4 Nearest Neighbor Classification

Nearest neighbor rules are simple nonparametric methods for classifying specimens that can capture nonlinearities in the true boundary between classes when the number of specimens is sufficient. Because the method does not involve estimation of numerous parameters, it often is an effective method even when the number of specimens is relatively small. A new specimen is classified based on the class labels of specimens in the training set to which its gene expression profile is most similar, or nearest (see Figure 8.2). A distance function or similarity measure is necessary for implementing the nearest neighbor method; common choices are Euclidean distance, Mahalanobis distance, and one minus the correlation coefficient. These distance measures are computed only with regard to the genes selected during the feature selection step.

The k-nearest neighbor method for classifying a specimen with unknown class label and expression profile vector $\mathbf{x}$ is as follows. Choose a distance function and use it to compute the distance between $\mathbf{x}$ and the gene expression profile of every specimen in the training set. Identify the k profiles in the training set closest to $\mathbf{x}$. The class of $\mathbf{x}$ is predicted to be the majority class

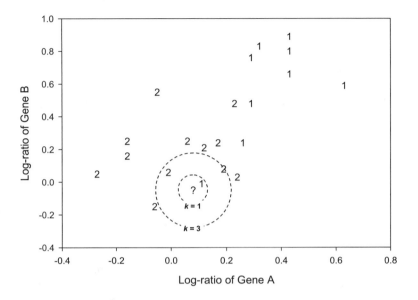

Fig. 8.2. Nearest neighbor analysis for prediction involving two classes. Specimens are represented in two-dimensional space based on expression of two selected genes of the profile (i.e., gene A and gene B). A **1** or **2** indicates specimens in class 1 or class 2, respectively. A new specimen to be classified is indicated by a **?**. For $k = 1$, the label of the nearest neighbor (using Euclidean distance) of the new specimen is 1, and this is the predicted class of the new specimen. For $k = 3$, the three nearest neighbors of the new specimen have labels of 1, 2, and 2; a simple majority rule results in the prediction of 2. In general, nearest neighbor classification is performed in more than two dimensions (i.e., using more than two genes).

label (or plurality class label if there are more than two classes) of its k nearest neighbors.

The number of neighbors k is usually chosen a priori. For small sample sizes, smaller values of k such as 1 or 3 are most appropriate. Li et al. (2001) were able to successfully classify colon tissue samples as normal or cancerous using a nearest neighbor rule with $k = 3$. Optimized values of k were generally less than 7 in the studies of Dudoit et al. (2002). Using an odd-valued k ensures no ties in two-class prediction.

8.3.5 Classification Trees

Classification trees have been used for classification of specimens using microarray gene expression profiles (Zhang et al. 2001; Dudoit et al. 2002).

Breiman et al. (1984) and Hastie et al. (2001) give comprehensive descriptions of classification tree methodology. Construction of a classification tree or, more specifically, a binary tree-structured classifier begins with a split of the gene expression profiles into two subsets (or nodes) based on the expression level of one of the genes; that is, one subset consists of those samples with expression level of the selected gene above a selected threshold value, and the other subset consists of the remaining samples. Ideally, the split is chosen to produce two subsets that are each homogeneous with regard to class labels. That is, one of the subsets will consist of specimens of class 1 and the other of specimens in class 2. Usually there will be no gene and threshold value that produces such an ideal split, and the split will be selected based on optimizing a function that measures class label homogeneity of the resulting two subsets.

After finding the gene and threshold value that optimally splits the set of samples of the training set into two subsets, the process is then repeated independently for each of the two resultant subsets. That is, for each of the subsets, the gene and threshold value that best separates the samples in that subset are determined. This process of binary splitting of subsets results in a tree structure. Each node of the tree represents a set of samples. Each node is split based on a gene and a threshold expression level.

The tree is grown in a hierarchical fashion until some stopping criterion is attained. A variety of stopping criteria are in use. For example, splitting of a node may cease if the samples represented by the node are sufficiently homogeneous with regard to class labels or if there are fewer than a specified number of samples in the node. The root node at the top of the tree contains all of the samples. Terminal nodes in the tree are assigned to a class. The class assigned to a terminal node may be simply the class most prevalent in the samples associated with that node. This majority rule may be modified to take into consideration different a priori probabilities for class membership or to take into account different costs of misclassification. For example, it may be more serious to misclassify a sample as class 2 when it is really class 1, than vice versa. The rule for assigning a class to each terminal node is the basis for the classification of new samples. Classification of a new specimen is then a simple matter determining in which terminal node the new specimen would be contained. The class of the unknown specimen is predicted to be the class assigned to that terminal node.

A simple classification tree is shown in Figure 8.3. Node 1 contains the entire dataset (20 gene expression profiles, 10 from each class). The first split is based on expression of gene A: profiles with a log ratio less than or equal to 1.4 form node 2 and the other profiles form node 3. Node 2 requires further partitioning due to the heterogeneity of specimens in this subset. Node 3, however, is sufficiently homogeneous to be a terminal node, assigned the prediction of class 1. A different gene (gene B) is used for the split of node 2 into daughter nodes: one of these (node 4) only contains specimens of class 2 and is thus a terminal node with a prediction of class 2, whereas the other (node 5) requires another split to reach satisfactory levels of purity for prediction.

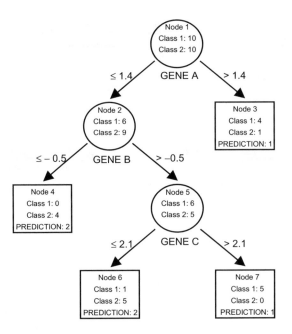

Fig. 8.3. A classification tree for prediction involving two classes: circles represent internal nodes that are further split; squares represent terminal nodes that are assigned a class prediction (indicated inside each square). The name under an internal node is the gene used for splitting that node; the numbers beside the arrows indicate the threshold value used for the split.

Perhaps the most important aspect of tree construction is the decision of when to stop splitting nodes. It is, of course, possible to keep making splits until all terminal nodes are completely pure, containing only specimens of one class. However, doing so is not recommended: continuing to split until absolute purity is attained likely results in overfitting the classification tree to the training set data. Trees created in such a fashion will have much poorer classification accuracy when applied to new specimens. To address this problem, Breiman et al. (1984) considered pruned versions of overgrown trees, selecting the best tree by a cross-validation approach. Another approach to lessen overfitting is to aggregate classification trees constructed from perturbed versions of the training set; this has been shown to lead to gains in classification accuracy (Breiman 1996, 1998).

8.3.6 Support Vector Machines

A *support vector machine* is a classification algorithm. Linear support vector machines attempt to find a linear combination of the features that best separates the specimens into two groups based on their class labels. When perfect separation is not possible, the optimal linear combination is determined by a criterion to minimize the number of misclassifications. For microarray data, linear support vector machine classification is based on a linear combination of log gene expression values. In this way it is similar to linear discriminant analysis, but the method of determining the weights of the linear combination is different. There are also many types of nonlinear support vector machines (Vapnik 1998), but to date there is little evidence that they are more effective than linear versions for gene expression data where the dimensionality of the data is very large relative to the number of samples. Support vector machines have also been used for the categorization of genes into functional classes (Brown 2000) and for the classification of ovarian tissue specimens as normal or cancerous (Furey 2000).

8.3.7 Comparison of Methods

Published studies of new prediction methods applied to microarray data are often of the proof-of-principle variety, using relatively easy classification problems (e.g., normal tissue versus cancer) and not making a comparison to established prediction methods. The lack of comparison to standard prediction methods is problematic: it is more interesting to see if the new method has an advantage over established methods than to see that the new method performs very well on an easy classification problem. This is not to say that an exhaustive comparison of prediction methods should be undertaken in order to determine the consensus best method for class prediction; no single method is likely to be optimal in all situations. The relative performance of methods is likely to depend on the biological classification under investigation, the genetic disparity among classes, within-class heterogeneity, and size of the training set.

Direct comparisons of class prediction methods can, however, provide valuable insight about which methods perform well under certain conditions. Dudoit et al. (2002) compared several of the methods described in this section: standard and diagonal discriminant analysis, Golub's weighted vote method, classification trees with and without aggregation, and nearest neighbor classification. The methods were applied to three microarray datasets: adult lymphoid malignancies separated into two or three classes (Alizadeh et al. 2000), acute lymphocytic and myelogenous leukemia (Golub et al. 1999), and sixty human tumor cell lines divided into eight classes based on site of origin (Ross et al. 2000). The genes selected for inclusion in the model were the G genes with the best univariate ability to discriminate the classes. They used $G = 30$ for the 60 cell line data, $G = 40$ for the leukemia dataset, and $G = 50$ for the lymphoma dataset.

Diagonal discriminant analysis and nearest neighbor classification had the best overall performance in the study. Classification trees had intermediate performance. Aggregation of classification trees tended to improve performance. Fisher linear discriminant analysis performed the worst. A distance measure that does not account for correlations between genes was used for nearest neighbor classification in the comparison performed by Dudoit et al. (2002). Thus the best performing methods in the study were those that ignored gene correlations and interactions. Moreover, the worst performing method (Fisher linear discriminant analysis) is one that explicitly incorporates gene correlation structure into class prediction. The authors did not select so many genes (G) that the linear discriminant model could not be fit, but still the number of correlation parameters that had to be estimated resulted in very poor predictive performance. The performance of Fisher linear discriminant analysis improved substantially when the number of included genes was limited to $G = 10$. The results of the comparison of methods do not necessarily indicate that correlations and interactions between genes are not important in the biological systems investigated. Rather, it is more likely that higher-level structure does exist in the underlying biological systems, but not enough information exists in the datasets studied to provide accurate estimates of this structure (the largest of the three datasets contained only 81 specimens). Class prediction methods that incorporate gene correlations and interactions are likely to become more useful as much larger gene expression datasets become available.

8.4 Estimating the Error Rate of the Predictor

8.4.1 Bias of the Re-Substitution Estimate

Using the same set of data for developing a predictive model and for evaluating the predictive accuracy of the model can result in a very biased overestimation of its predictive accuracy. The reason is that the parameters of the model are optimized to fit the dataset and they will fit those data better than they will predict for independent data. This phenomenon is called overfitting. For traditional kinds of statistical modeling with many cases and few parameters, the degree of bias may not be severe. But when the number of parameters is orders of magnitude greater than the number of cases (specimens), the degree of bias can be huge. For gene expression data, each candidate gene might be used in the predictive model and thus represents a parameter. As noted above, even once a relatively small number of genes are selected in the feature selection step for inclusion in the prediction model, the number of parameters available for fitting that model to the data may easily exceed the number of specimens.

Simon et al. (2003) illustrated the bias of the conventional *resubstitution estimate* of misclassification rate for DNA microarray data. The resubstitution estimate is calculated by using the dataset to select variables and fit the predictive model, then using the model to predict class membership for the same specimens, counting the number of errors made. Simon et al. (2003) generated simulated data for measuring expression levels on 6000 genes for each of 20 specimens. The data were generated randomly, using the same Gaussian distribution for each gene and each specimen. After generating the random data, specimens 1 through 10 were arbitrarily considered to be from class 1 and specimens 11 through 20 from class 2. They utilized the entire 20 specimens for feature selection to identify the 10 genes that were most differentially expressed between the two classes, and then developed the simple compound covariate predictor described in Section 8.3.3.2 based on these selected genes. Having developed the model, they predicted the class of each of the 20 specimens and counted the number of misclassification errors of this resubstitution estimate. They repeated this procedure for 2000 randomly simulated datasets, and the results are shown in Figure 8.4. It was found that

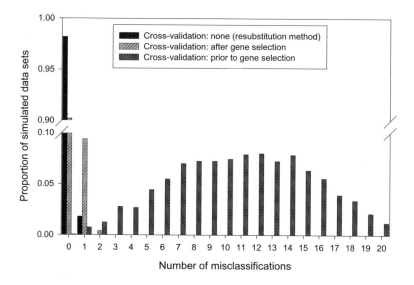

Fig. 8.4. The effect of various levels of cross-validation on the estimated error rate of a predictor. Two thousand datasets were simulated as described in the text. Class labels were arbitrarily assigned to the specimens within each dataset, so poor classification accuracy is expected. Class prediction was performed on each dataset as described in the text, varying the level of leave-one-out cross-validation used in prediction. Vertical bars indicate the proportion of simulated datasets (out of 2000) resulting in a given number of misclassifications for a specified cross-validation strategy. Adapted from Simon et al. (2003).

98.2% of the datasets resulted in a resubstitution estimate of zero errors, even though no true difference existed between the two classes. Moreover, the maximum number of misclassified specimens using the resubstitution estimate was only one.

8.4.2 Cross-Validation and Bootstrap Estimates of Error Rate

Ultimately, the goal is to construct a classifier that will accurately predict class labels for new specimens not involved in the creation of the prediction rule. Methods are available to estimate the true error rate of the predictor (i.e., the probability of incorrectly classifying a randomly selected future case) with much less bias than the resubstitution estimate. One commonly used method is cross-validation. Cross-validation is accomplished by leaving out a portion of the specimens, building the prediction rule on the remaining specimens, referred to as the *training set*, and predicting the class labels of the left-out specimens. *Leave-one-out cross-validation* is a common choice for the small sample sizes commonly encountered in microarray studies (see Figure 8.5). Each specimen is left-out, one at a time. For each training set with one specimen left out, feature selection is performed from scratch and a predictive model is built. That model is then used to predict the class of the left-out specimen. That prediction is then counted as being correct or incorrect. The entire procedure is repeated for each specimen left out and the total number of classification errors is determined (Hills 1966; Lachenbruch and Mickey 1968).

There is considerable confusion about leave-one-out cross-validation. Many investigators do not appreciate the importance of repeatedly performing feature selection for each leave-one-out training set. In fact, feature selection is frequently the most important part of model development. With good features, the particular form of the model is often not crucial. However, this means that failing to cross-validate feature selection is a failure to remove a major source of bias in the resubstitution estimate. In our simulations of class prediction of random classes, we examined the bias in estimated error rates for class prediction with various levels of cross-validation (Simon et al. 2003). Two types of leave-one-out cross-validation were considered: one repeating feature selection of differentially expressed genes for each leave-one-out training set, and one in which feature selection of univariately informative genes is performed using the entire dataset before starting the cross-validation. In the latter case, the same set of genes is used to build the model for each leave-one-out step, although the weights of the genes vary from step to step.

Figure 8.4 shows the observed number of misclassifications resulting from each level of cross-validation for 2000 simulated datasets. The true misclassification rate should be 50% because the classes are random. As shown in the figure, 98.2% of the simulated datasets resulted in a resubstitution estimate of zero misclassifications. Improper cross-validation without repeating feature selection for each training set led to very biased low estimates of the

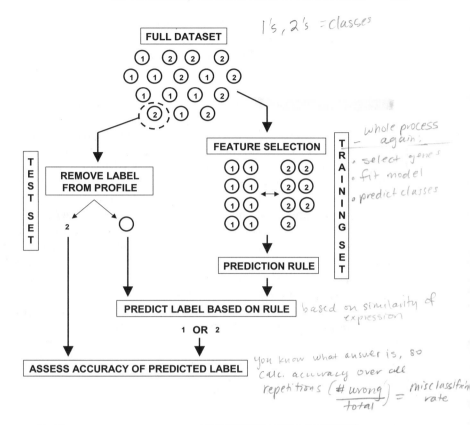

Fig. 8.5. A single step of the leave-one-out method of cross-validation. A single specimen is removed from the full dataset. The left-out specimen is the *test set* and the remaining specimens comprise the *training set* for the step. Feature selection is performed on the training set in a supervised fashion (i.e., comparing class 1 to class 2) and a prediction rule is built from the selected features. The prediction rule is applied to the gene expression profile of the left-out specimen (which has been stripped of its class label) and the correctness of this prediction is noted. A leave-one-out step is performed for every specimen in the full dataset.

misclassification (Figure 8.4): 90.2 % of simulated datasets still result in zero misclassifications. When gene selection is also subjected to cross-validation, then the prediction results match expectation: the median number of misclassified profiles jumps to 11 (the true misclassification rate is 50% or 10 misclassified profiles).

   Data imputation will frequently be necessary during cross-validation, as missing data are common in microarray studies (see Chapter 5 for a discussion of imputation methods). As mentioned in Section 8.2, imputation should be avoided prior to the feature selection step, if possible. This means imputation takes place after feature selection within each leave-one-out step of the cross-validation procedure. Imputation of missing values for the left-out specimen is not suggested, or necessary. Instead, all selected features for which the left-out specimen has a missing value should simply be omitted from the prediction rule. Imputation is only necessary for a training set specimen that has a missing selected feature that is not missing for the left-out specimen.

Bootstrap estimation of the true error rate is an alternative to cross-validation. Bootstrapping is accomplished by selecting, with replacement, n specimens from among the original set of n specimens. Sampling with replacement means that some specimens may be present multiple times in the bootstrap sample. A predictive model is developed from scratch on the bootstrap sample. "From scratch" means not forgetting to repeat the gene selection step for the bootstrap sample. The model is then used to predict what class each of the specimens not in the bootstrap sample belongs to and each prediction is recorded as correct or incorrect. This entire process is repeated for many bootstrap samples and the average number of misclassifications per prediction is used as an estimate of the misclassification rate. An advantage of bootstrap estimates, especially for small sample sizes, is that they have smaller variances than estimates derived from leave-one-out cross-validation. These simple bootstrap estimates tend to have bias, but more complex bootstrapping procedures with less bias have been proposed (Efron and Tibshirani 1997). More extensive descriptions of error rate estimation by bootstrapping are given by Efron (1983) and Efron and Tibshirani (1998). Cross validation procedures that omit more than a single observation at a time may also reduce the variance of the estimated error rate.

8.4.3 Reporting Error Rates

Investigators should not report the resubstitution estimate of the misclassification rate. It only serves to encourage misinterpretation. Furthermore, estimates of the error rate should incorporate results for all specimens examined. Some predictors allow a specimen to remain unclassified if the specimen cannot confidently be assigned to any of the examined classes. For example, the weighted vote method (Golub et al. 1999) assigns a prediction strength index to each sample. Specimens may be assigned to an uncertain class if the absolute value of the prediction strength index for a specimen does not exceed a specified threshold. Although "uncertain" may be a clinically important category, it may also be seen as a failure of the classification procedure. Simply ignoring unclassified specimens in the estimation of the true error rate gives an overly optimistic impression. For example, a classifier that classifies one sample correctly and calls the rest uncertain has 100% accuracy by disregarding unclassified specimens but at the same time is of little practical value. The correct classification rate (number correctly classified out of the total examined) and the misclassification rate (number misclassified out of the total examined) seem the most pertinent statistics.

8.4.4 Statistical Significance of the Error Rate

In addition to obtaining an unbiased estimate of the misclassification rate, it is also possible to determine whether the estimate is statistically significantly lower than what one would expect by chance for two classes that did not really differ with regard to the gene expression profile. This can be useful because it is possible in some cases to achieve a relatively small error rate estimate even for random data. For example, in the simulation described above, more than 12% of the datasets resulted in five or fewer correctly cross-validated misclassifications (an error rate of $\leq 25\%$) even though expression profiles for the two classes were generated from the same distribution. Radmacher et al. (2002) proposed the use of a permutation method to assess the statistical significance of a cross-validated error rate. The probability of producing a cross-validated error rate as small as that observed given no association between class membership and the expression profiles is estimated by a permutation test, and this estimate serves as the achieved significance level (i.e., p-value). Under the null hypothesis that no systematic difference in gene expression profiles exists between the two classes, it can be assumed that assignment of gene expression profiles to class labels is purely coincidental (Lehmann and Stein 1949). This situation is mimicked by randomly permuting labels among the gene expression profiles. For each random permutation of class labels, the entire leave-one-out cross-validation procedure is performed to estimate a cross-validated misclassification rate. This is repeated for a large number of random permutations of the class labels. Thus one estimates the distribution of the cross-validated misclassification rate under the null hypothesis that there is no relation between class and gene expression profile.

Ideally, an exact permutation test would be performed, examining every possible permutation of the class labels. In practice this is burdensome due to the large number of permutations for even modest sample sizes. Radmacher et al. (2002) suggest that using 2000 random permutations is sufficient.

8.4.5 Validation Dataset

Using cross-validation or bootstrap sampling to estimate the misclassification rate requires that there be some defined algorithm for gene selection and model building that can be automatically applied within each leave-one-out or bootstrap sample training set. For some studies this is not the case because many methods are tried during the analysis and some steps of the analysis depend on findings in previous steps in a manner that is not easily specified in an algorithmic manner. For such studies, it is best to separate the data into a training set and a validation set before any analysis takes place. The validation set is locked away and not used until a single completely specified predictive model is developed on the training data. At that time, the completely specified model is applied to the specimens in the validation set to predict to which class each of those specimens belongs, and the misclassification rate is computed.

Rosenwald et al. (2002) used this approach for the development of a prognostic index for patients with large B-cell lymphomas.

In using the split sample approach, a plan for splitting the sample into training and validation subsets is needed. Rosenwald et al. (2002) used two thirds of their data for the training set. The training set is used for identifying the genes to include in the predictive model and for developing a completely specified model, including the estimation of model parameters; the validation set is used only to calculate the predictive accuracy of the model. Consequently, it is reasonable to assign the majority of the specimens to the training set. It is best to determine in advance how many specimens will be required for each set.

Very small datasets, containing 10 or fewer specimens, are often used for validation of a predictor, but such small datasets are really inadequate. For example, MacDonald et al. (2001) built a predictor from the gene expression profiles of 23 medulloblastoma specimens that distinguished between metastatic and nonmetastatic cases; the predictor had good cross-validated prediction accuracy on the training set (72% correctly classified). An additional dataset consisting of expression data for four tumors was analyzed and the predictor correctly classified the four new tumors. This was interpreted as a preliminary confirmation of the results. However, the 95% confidence bounds on the true error rate derived from the independent validation study are 0 to 53%. Thus, even with perfect classification of the independent specimens, it cannot be stated with confidence that prediction is better than a fifty-fifty guess. The validation set should also contain a sufficient number of tumors of each class.

8.5 Example

To illustrate several of the methods described in this chapter we use the 22 expression profiles of breast tumors reported by Hedenfalk et al. (2001). These tumors were classified with regard to whether they were obtained from women with germline BRCA1 or BRCA2 mutations. The data are described in Appendix B. Seven of the tumors were from women with germline BRCA1 mutations, eight were from women with germline BRCA2 mutations, and seven contained neither germline mutation. We developed classifiers for distinguishing tumors from women with BRCA2 mutations from the other 14 tumors. Data were available for the 3226 genes that were considered well measured on the arrays by the original investigators. We developed classifiers based on Fisher linear discriminant analysis (FLDA), diagonal linear discriminant analysis (DLDA), compound covariate predictor (CCP), support vector machine with linear kernel (SVM), k-nearest neighbor predictors with k equal to 1 and 3, and classification trees (CART). For feature selection we used the genes that were univariately statistically significant at a stringent $p < 0.001$ significance level using the t-test to compare log expression ratios in the two classes. Features were reselected for each leave-one-out cross-validation training set.

For Fisher linear discriminant analysis we utilized no more than five genes in the feature selection set, however, because using the full set of significant genes gave noninvertible covariance matrices. This is an inherent limitation of Fisher linear discriminant analysis.

We used leave-one-out cross-validation (LOOCV) to evaluate the misclassification rate for each type of classifier. Consequently we developed classifiers of each type for all of the 22 training sets obtained by omitting samples one at a time. We computed the t-tests, selected the genes to be included in the model, and fit the model from scratch for each of the 22 training sets. Table 8.1 shows the results of prediction for each classifier and each of the 22 training sets.

Table 8.1. Cross-Validated Correct Classification Rates

Sample Removed	BRCA2 Mutation	Correct Prediction?						
		DLDA	CCP	FLDA	1-NN	3-NN	SVM	CART
1900	+	no	no	no	yes	no	no	no
1787	+	yes	yes	yes	yes	yes	no	yes
1721	+	yes	yes	yes	yes	yes	yes	no
1486	+	no	no	no	yes	no	yes	no
1816	+	yes	yes	yes	yes	yes	yes	yes
1616	+	yes	yes	yes	yes	no	yes	no
1063	+	yes	yes	yes	yes	yes	yes	yes
1936	+	yes	yes	no	yes	yes	yes	no
1996	−	yes	yes	yes	yes	yes	yes	yes
1822	−	yes	yes	no	yes	yes	yes	yes
1714	−	yes	yes	yes	yes	yes	yes	yes
1224	−	yes	yes	no	yes	yes	yes	yes
1252	−	yes	yes	no	no	no	no	no
1510	−	yes	yes	yes	yes	yes	yes	yes
1572	−	yes	yes	no	yes	yes	yes	no
1324	−	no	no	no	no	no	no	yes
1649	−	yes	yes	yes	yes	yes	yes	no
1320	−	yes	yes	yes	yes	yes	yes	no
1542	−	yes	yes	yes	yes	yes	yes	no
1281	−	yes	yes	yes	yes	yes	yes	yes
1321	−	yes	yes	yes	yes	yes	yes	yes
1905	−	yes	yes	yes	yes	yes	yes	yes
Correct Classification		86%	86%	64%	91%	77%	82%	55%

We begin with a discussion of the four related methods. Diagonal linear discriminant analysis and the compound covariate predictor had 86% correct cross-validated prediction. Each had three prediction errors, two for BRCA2 positive cases and one for a BRCA2 negative case. They predicted correctly and incorrectly for exactly the same set of cases. Fisher linear discriminant analysis did not do as well, having only 64% correct cross-validated prediction. It predicted incorrectly for the same three cases as did DLDA and CPP, but it predicted incorrectly for an additional five BRCA2 negative cases. The support vector machine with linear kernel had four cross-validated misclassifications for an 82% correct prediction rate.

Figure 8.6 shows the weights assigned to individual genes for the linear methods DLDA, CPP, and SVM plotted against each other. There were 49 genes statistically significant at the $p < 0.001$ level by t-test for the complete set of 22 samples and so the graphs in Figure 8.6 each contain 49 points. These weights are based on fitting the models to the complete set of 22 samples. (Although FLDA is also a linear method, it utilized only 5 genes and so it is not shown in the figure.) The figure indicates that the weights for the different methods have the same sign but different values. The set of selected genes varied for each leave-one-out training set, therefore we examined how frequently each of these 49 genes had a $p < 0.001$ in the 22 leave-one-out training sets. If we rank these 49 genes based on their p values for the full set of 22 samples, we find that the 24 genes with the smallest overall p-values had p-values of less than 0.001 in all of the 22 training sets. The 9 genes with the next smallest overall p-values had p-values less than 0.001 in 15 to 20 of the training sets. The remaining genes had p-values of less than 0.001 in only 3 to12 of the training sets. This type of information is helpful in evaluating the importance of individual genes in the final model fit to the full data.

The 1-nearest neighbor classification method had only two cross-validated misclassifications for a correct prediction rate of 91%. It classified all of the BRCA2 cases correctly and misclassified two BRCA2 negative cases. The 3-nearest neighbor method had five misclassifications, including three of the BRCA2 cases, for a correct prediction rate of 77%.

The CART classification tree did very poorly, achieving a correct cross-validated prediction rate of only 55%. This is approximately the rate one would expect if one predicted randomly based on the proportion of BRCA2 specimens in the leave-one-out training sets. The tree classifier approach might have done better had we employed some of the "bagging" and "boosting" strategies for averaging different tree classifiers as described in Dudoit et al. (2002).

The classification tree approach tends to place great weight on expression levels for single genes. This makes for nice interpretability and ease of clinical implementation. Unfortunately, it tends to give inaccurate predictions when there are limited numbers of cases. It is too easy to find single genes or pairs of genes that are highly predictive of outcome for any training set but which are useless for classifying new specimens. In data-limited settings, methods that base classification on averaging expression for larger numbers of genes tend to perform better.

For illustration, we applied the CART classification tree algorithm to the complete dataset of 22 samples using the genes statistically significant at

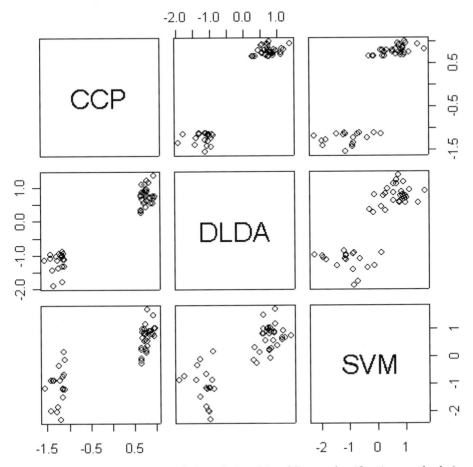

Fig. 8.6. Scatterplot matrix of the relationship of linear classification methods in the weights they placed on expression levels of individual genes for the example of Section 8.5: CCP denotes the compound covariate predictor, DLDA denotes diagonal linear discriminant analysis, and SVM denotes the support vector machine with linear kernel. Each panel of the matrix shows a scatterplot comparing two linear classification methods. Each point on a scatterplot represents a gene used for classification by the methods. For each method, the weights have been standardized to have mean zero and standard deviation one.

the $p < 0.001$ level for the complete data as candidate predictors. The tree selected by the algorithm used only one candidate predictor and had only two terminal nodes. The probe used had Image clone identifier 51209 and an annotation of "Protein phosphatase 1, catalytic subunit, beta isoform." The optimal threshold for classification based on that probe was a log ratio value of 0.029. Samples with log ratios for this clone of less than 0.029 were classified as BRCA2 mutated; samples with log ratios for this clone greater than the threshold were classified as not BRCA2 mutated. In the full dataset, nine samples had log ratios less than the threshold and eight of them carried germline BRCA2 mutations. Consequently, there is only one misclassification in the complete dataset for the model developed using the complete data. Obviously, this estimate of misclassification rate is highly biased, as seen from the cross-validation results.

8.6 Prognostic Prediction

Some microarray studies are designed to determine whether there is a relationship between expression profile and clinical outcome and to develop a prognostic predictor of outcome based on the level of expression of selected genes. Sometimes outcome is categorical. For example, some pharmacogenomic studies attempt to distinguish between patients who will and will not experience toxicity to an effective treatment for a disease. The research objective in such a study can be considered a two-group class prediction as discussed above. In many studies, however, outcome is not categorical. One example is a study of clinical outcome in patients with diffuse large B-cell lymphoma (Rosenwald et al. 2002). In that study a prognostic model was developed for predicting duration of patient survival, with continuous right-censored outcome data. The prediction methods described previously in this chapter cannot be directly applied to such data.

For survival studies one may evaluate the association of the expression level of a gene i with survival by fitting a proportional hazards regression model containing only the gene i expression values as described in Section 7.8. For such a model, the statistical significance test of the null hypothesis of no association between survival and the expression of gene i can be based on a statistic z_i which under the null hypothesis has a standard Gaussian distribution with mean zero and standard deviation one. These tests can be performed for all genes, and those genes with their z_i values sufficiently great in absolute value can be selected for multivariate modeling.

In analogy to the compound covariate predictor for class prediction, we can form a prognostic index for survival as a weighted sum of expression measures for genes with univariate prognostic significance in the dataset. The prognostic index for specimen j is

$$c_j = \sum_{i=1}^{G} z_j x_{ji}, \tag{8.13}$$

where z_i is a standardized Gaussian statistic for selected gene i and x_{ji} is the log expression measurement of selected gene i in specimen j. The summation is over only the genes selected based on the magnitude of their z values. The prognostic index has the same form as the compound covariate predictor (Equation (8.10)), but with different weights.

The prognostic index (8.13) can be used to classify the patients into good and poor risk groups. Leave-one-out cross-validation can be used to estimate the difference in survival distributions of the predicted risk groups. Prognosis groups can be formed in the leave-one-out training set based on values of the c_j. For example, having computed the z_i values for all genes and selected the genes to be used for computing the prognostic index, compute c_j values for all specimens in the training set and for the specimen left out. If the c_j value for the specimen left-out is smaller than the median c_j value of the specimens in the training set, then the left out specimen is predicted to be from a good prognosis patient. Otherwise, the specimen left out is predicted to be from a poor prognosis patient. This is because in the analysis of proportional hazards models, large values of the regression coefficients are associated with a poor prognosis. This entire process of gene selection, prognostic index computation, and prediction of prognosis for the left-out specimen is repeated for each leave-one-out training set.

Having predicted a prognostic group for each specimen in a fully cross-validated manner, the Kaplan Meier survival curves of these two prognostic groups can be computed and graphed (Lawless 1982). The difference between these survival curves is an unbiased estimate of the effect of prognostic classification using a gene expression-based prognostic index.

There will often be interest in establishing whether the survival distributions for the prognostic groups are different. The usual statistical tests for comparing the Kaplan Meier survival curves are not valid because the groups were not prespecified independently of the survival data. Consequently, a permutation analysis is needed to test statistical significance. We start by computing a standard statistic for the two survival curves obtained from the analysis of the data, for example, the log-rank statistic. Call this value LR*. We then randomly permute the survival times (and associated censoring indicators) among specimens. We then repeat the entire cross-validation procedure described above, obtaining two new prognostic groups, two new Kaplan Meier survival curves, and a new value of the log-rank test comparing these two new survival curves. By redoing this process with a large number of random permutations of the survival times, we generate the distribution of log-rank values under the null hypothesis that there is no association between survival and gene expression profile. The proportion of these random permutations that give good and poor risk groups properly ordered and a log-rank value at least as large as the value LR* for the real data is the p-value associated with a test of the null hypothesis.

9

Class Discovery

9.1 Introduction

In this chapter we discuss methods useful for discovering patterns in microarray data. More specifically, we focus on methods of identifying groups of co-expressed genes, and for finding patterns in the expression profiles of different specimens when there is no predefined class variable to supervise the analysis. Patterns may consist of a classification into subgroupings, or clusters, and there may be multilevel structure within the classification. *Cluster analysis* techniques can be applied to construct classifications of specimens or experimental conditions (arrays), or they can be applied to construct classifications of genes; sometimes they are applied to construct classifications on the two dimensions simultaneously. For example, using a cluster analysis technique known as *hierarchical clustering*, Alizadeh et al. (2000) discovered new subgroups of lymphomas. Similarly, Bittner et al. (2000) found structure among otherwise morphologically indistinguishable melanoma tumors. Tamayo et al. (1999) used microarrays to study gene expression in HL-60 cells and uncovered several biologically interesting clusters of genes involved in hematopoietic differentiation using a clustering technique known as *self-organizing maps* (SOMs). For the analysis methods discussed here, no supplemental information need accompany the specimens or genes to suggest existing structure or classification; therefore, they fall into the category of *unsupervised methods.*

Visualization of microarray data by means of graphical displays can be very helpful in discovering patterns in microarray expression profiles. Some of the graphical displays we discuss are specific to certain cluster analysis methods, and others are generic methods of representing high-dimensional data in lower dimensions. Examples of displays linked to a specific clustering algorithm include clustering trees called *dendrograms* and color image plots, both of which are ways of representing results of a hierarchical clustering. *Multidimensional scaling* is an example of a generic display method.

In the discussion and examples of this chapter, it is assumed that data preprocessing has already been conducted along the lines described in Chap-

ters 4 through 6. Definitions of distance and similarity measures, which are
at the core of many cluster analysis algorithms, are covered in Section 9.2.
Generic graphical display methods are described in Section 9.3. Graphical displays linked to a specific clustering algorithm are discussed in the section in
which the algorithm is defined. We discuss specific clustering methods in Section 9.4. Cluster analysis methods can be powerful exploratory tools, but it is
important to bear in mind that clustering algorithms can detect clusters even
on random data. Therefore, an assessment of the validity of putative clusters
is essential. The assessment should be based both on biological plausibility
and level of statistical evidence for clusters. In Section 9.5 we discuss several
statistically based methods for assessing clustering results.

9.2 Similarity and Distance Metrics

Most clustering methods are based on some measure of similarity or distance
(dissimilarity) defined between objects, with the goal being to group together
similar objects. When considering a *distance* or *dissimilarity metric*, it is understood that the larger the calculated value, the greater the difference between objects. Larger values of a *similarity metric* represent more similar
objects. *Euclidean distance, Manhattan distance, Mahalanobis distance, angular distance*, and *Pearson correlation* are the bases for some of the most
common distance and similarity metrics. Several measures of similarity or
dissimilarity between two arrays are defined below. Let x_{j_1} denote a vector of
the log expression levels for all of the genes on the array numbered j_1, that
is, $x_{j_1} = (x_{j_1 1}, x_{j_1 2}, \ldots, x_{j_1 K})$, where K denotes the number of genes on the
array. Similarly, let x_{j_2} denote the vector of log expression levels for the array
numbered j_2, and thus $x_{j_2} = (x_{j_2 1}, x_{j_2 2}, \ldots, x_{j_2 K})$. Similarity or dissimilarity
measures between two genes are defined analogously by reversing the roles
of arrays and genes in each of the calculations described below. To avoid the
laborious presentation of the measures for both arrays and genes, we present
them only for the case of measuring similarity or dissimilarity between arrays.
Euclidean distance between profiles from two arrays is computed by calculating for each gene the difference in its expression values between the two
arrays, summing the squares of those differences over all genes, and then taking the square root of that sum. Sometimes weights are applied to the squared
differences by multiplying each squared difference by a weight prior to summing over the genes, and then the result is a weighted Euclidean distance. One
might wish to use a weighted distance when expression values are missing for
some genes on some arrays. If one pair of arrays has fewer gene expression
measurements available for both arrays than does another pair of arrays, then
the distance between the arrays of pair one and the distance between the
arrays of pair two are not directly comparable. To make the distances more
comparable, one might sum over the nonmissing genes and use a weight for
every gene that is the reciprocal of the number of genes for which expression

values are available for both arrays. This weighted distance corresponds to a root mean squared difference. (Alternatively, one could have imputed values for the missing measurements instead of using a weighted distance.)

Mahalanobis distance is another type of weighted distance measure. The idea behind it is to downweight contributions of genes with large variance and contributions of genes that are highly correlated with other genes. A difficulty in using it when clustering arrays is that it cannot be calculated if the number of genes exceeds that number of arrays, a typical situation. However, this distance measure could be considered when clustering genes.

Manhattan distance (sometimes called the city block metric) between profiles from two arrays is computed by calculating for each gene the absolute difference in its expression values between the two arrays and summing those absolute differences over all genes. A weighted version can also be used. The advantage of Manhattan distance over Euclidean distance is its robustness to extreme observations. As a result of the squaring of the difference terms in Euclidean distance, it particularly heavily weights large differences, whereas the Manhattan distance will be less influenced by these extreme differences. In a comparison of clustering methods and distance metrics, Rahnenfuehrer (2002) found the Manhattan distance to be one of the best performers.

Pearson correlation computed between the expression measurements from arrays j_1 and j_2 is a similarity metric that measures how well the expression measurements obtained on one of the arrays can be expressed as a linear function (i.e., multiplied by some constant value and shifted by some constant value) of the expression measurements on the other array. It is defined as

$$\frac{\sum_{k=1}^{K} \left(x_{j_1 k} - \bar{x}_{j_1} \right) \left(x_{j_2 k} - \bar{x}_{j_2} \right)}{\left(\sum_{k_1=1}^{K} \left(x_{j_1 k_1} - \bar{x}_{j_1} \right)^2 \sum_{k_2=1}^{K} \left(x_{j_2 k_2} - \bar{x}_{j_2} \right)^2 \right)^{1/2}}$$

where $\bar{x}_j$ is the mean expression measure over all genes on array j. Two profiles can be very dissimilar by Euclidean distance, yet be very similar by a correlation measure. For example, if the log expression level of each gene in specimen j_1 is exactly twice its expression level in specimen j_2, the correlation would take on its maximum value of one, but the two specimens would be very dissimilar by Euclidean distance because their absolute distance is large. Commonly used conventions to convert a correlation similarity metric to a distance metric are to take distance $= 1 -$ correlation, or to take distance $= (1 -$ correlation$)/2$. The latter option produces a distance between 0 and 1.

A more robust measure of correlation, such as *Spearman correlation* could also be used. The Spearman rank correlation is defined like the Pearson correlation except that within each profile, each gene expression measurement is replaced by its rank within that profile, and it is those ranks that are used in computing the correlation. The Spearman correlation is less sensitive to outlying observations and therefore tends to be more stable, but this stability can also come at the expense of some sensitivity to true patterns in the data. Also, it is not clear how to handle assignment of ranks if there are some missing expression measurements.

The uncentered version of the Pearson correlation, sometimes called angular distance, is

$$
\frac{\sum_{k=1}^{K} x_{j_1 k} x_{j_2 k}}{\left(\sum_{k_1=1}^{K} x_{j_1 k_1}^2 \sum_{k_2=1}^{K} x_{j_2 k_2}^2 \right)^{1/2}}
$$

It differs from the Pearson correlation in that there is no centering by subtraction of $\bar{x}_{j_1}$ and $\bar{x}_{j_2}$ from the expression measurements. It is called angular distance because it equals the cosine of the angle formed by the vectors that represent the arrays in K-dimensional space. Each array can be viewed as representing a point in K-dimensional space, and its vector representation is the vector that extends from the origin (all K coordinates equal to zero) to that point. As with the Pearson correlation, it is always between minus 1 and 1, and it can be transformed in a similar fashion to produce a distance between 0 and 1.

One additional point to note is that similarity and distance metrics must be interpreted in the context of any standardization or normalization that has been applied previously to the data. For example, if arrays have been normalized by subtracting the median across all genes, the angular distance will frequently approximate the Pearson correlation.

Another data preprocessing step that is often applied prior to clustering microarray data is mean or median centering of genes. For cDNA microarray data, this involves subtracting from each expression measurement for a given gene, the mean or median for that gene across the arrays. This centering removes the dependence of the ratios on the amount of expression of each gene in the reference sample; Table 9.1 demonstrates a simple example.

Table 9.1.

		Reference Sample	Test Sample 1	Test Sample 2
Gene 1	Expression intensity	200	400	800
	Expression ratio		2	4
	Log$_2$ (ratio)		1	2
	Centered[a] log$_2$ (ratio)		−0.5	0.5
Gene 2	Expression intensity	100	800	400
	Expression ratio		8	4
	Log$_2$ (ratio)		3	2
	Centered[b] log$_2$ (ratio)		0.5	−0.5

[a]Median (or mean) log$_2$(ratio) for gene 1 across two samples is 1.5.
[b]Median (or mean) log$_2$(ratio) for gene 2 across two samples is 2.5.

(Assume that the intensity measures in the table have already been adjusted for dye effects.) The true expression of gene 1 in sample 1 (400) and gene 2 in sample 2 (400) are the same, but because the two genes are represented in different amounts (200 versus 100) in the reference sample, the log ratios associated with them are not the same. By median centering, the (centered) log ratios are made the same for the two genes. In the example in Table 9.1, the median and mean are equivalent. In general, the median is a better choice than the mean because it will be less sensitive to a few potentially spurious extremely high or low expression measurements. Centering can also be performed on expression measurements besides log ratios, for example, expression levels from oligonucleotide arrays, because it serves as a type of standardization. The centering puts all genes on an equal footing and does not allow genes that tend to be very highly expressed to dominate distance metrics, and hence the behavior of the clustering algorithms. Note that if one is computing Euclidean distance between profiles for two specimens, this gene centering has no effect on the distance, because it subtracts out in the calculation. However, if one were computing Euclidean distance between two genes' profiles rather than between two specimens' profiles, this gene centering could have a very large impact on the resulting distance.

We tend to think of correlation of patterns as biologically relevant, and the absolute closeness required for small Euclidean distance often feels overly stringent. For this reason, we have more often used correlation-based similarity metrics or metrics that involve some scaling or standardization of expression measures. In general, the choice of similarity or dissimilarity metric needs to be made on a case-by-case basis.

9.3 Graphical Displays

9.3.1 Classical Multidimensional Scaling

The extremely high-dimensional nature of microarray data makes it impossible to visualize plots of array profiles or gene profiles unless they are represented in lower dimensions. Typically, two or three-dimensional displays are used. Multidimensional scaling is a very useful display technique that has been applied for the analysis of microarray data (see e.g, Khan et al. 1998 and Assersohn et al. 2002). We describe it here in the context of producing a display of J arrays. Classical multidimensional scaling addresses the following problem. Given a set of J points in a K-dimensional space, find a set of points (coordinates) in an s-dimensional space with $s < K$ such that the Euclidean distances between those points in the new space provide a good approximation to the distances between points in the original higher-dimensional space.

We begin with a simplified explanation of the related subject of *principal components analysis*. For multidimensional data, principal components analysis is a method for expressing data in a new coordinate system by finding weighted combinations of the original variables that have maximum variance and are constrained to be uncorrelated with one another (Hotelling 1933). These optimal weighted combinations are called principal components. Geometrically, if one visualizes a cloud of points in high-dimensional space, this involves a rigid rotation and translation (shifting) of the cloud of points so that the longest axis of the cloud is aligned with the first variable axis, and the next longest axis perpendicular to that first axis is aligned with the second variable axis, and so forth. It can be shown that the first s principal components satisfy the multidimensional scaling goal described above (Gordon 1999). It is also possible to calculate the proportion of the total variation in the data that is explained by the s-dimensional representation, and this proportion is sometimes used as a measure of the adequacy of the s-dimensional representation.

Figure 9.1 gives an example of a principal components transformation of some hypothetical three-dimensional data. The $\times$ and o symbols in the figure represent some underlying subclasses. In the top plot (panel (a), there is a single elliptical wafer with no thickness, oriented on an incline in three-dimensional space. Because this wafer has no thickness, it really occupies only a two-dimensional subspace. When we consider the two-dimensional principal components plot as shown in the lower plot (b), we see that no information has been lost in reducing to two dimensions, and the proportion of variance explained is 100%. Even if the wafer had had some uniform thickness, there would have been no information loss in reducing to two principal compnents regarding the comparison of the $\times$ symbols to the o symbols.

Figure 9.2 gives another example of a principal components transformation of some hypothetical three-dimensional data with two subclasses denoted by the $\times$ and o symbols. In the top of the figure (a), two thick elliptical wafers, lying one above the other, are oriented on an incline in three-dimensional space. The longest ("major") axis of the ellipse is length 8, and the shortest ("minor") axis of the ellipse is 4. (The short axis cannot readily be seen in the orientation of the axes pictured in Figure 9-2.) The thickness of each wafer is 0.4. The middle figure (b) shows the principal components transformation, that is, the three-dimensional plot of the principal components. Now the point cloud is centered at the intersection of the PC1, PC2, and PC3 axes. The major (longest) axis of the ellipse is aligned with the PC1 axis, the minor axis (perpendicular to the major axis) of the ellipse is aligned with the PC2 axis, and the thickness of the layered ellipses is in the direction of the PC3 axis. If we wanted a (lower) two-dimensional representation of these data points, we could consider plotting only the first two principal components as in the bottom figure (c). We would then completely lose the separation of the $\times$ symbols (top wafer) from the o symbols (bottom wafer). Interestingly, the proportion of variance explained by the two-dimensional projection is an impressive-sounding 98%, but because the important information that separated the wafers (each wafer corresponding to a subclass in this case) happened to be on the dimension of smallest variance, all of the critical in-

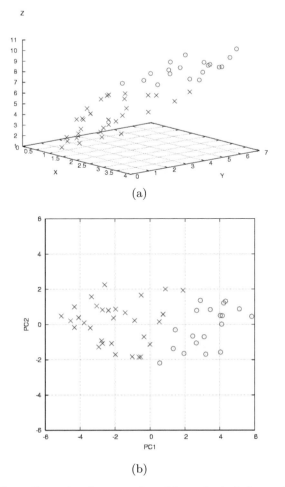

Fig. 9.1. (a) Three-dimensional scatterplot of hypothetical data arising from two subclasses denoted by × and o plotting symbols, (b) two-dimensional principal components representation of the data displayed in (a).

formation for distinguishing the two subclasses was lost when reducing from three to two dimensions.

Figure 9.3 presents a three-dimensional scaling display of log expression ratio profiles obtained from cDNA microarray assays performed on 31 melanoma tumors (Bittner et al. 2000) using a common reference design. Used in this analysis were the 3613 genes that were considered "strongly detected." Prior to the multidimensional scaling analysis, ratios greater than 50 or less than 0.02 were truncated at 50 and 0.02, respectively. More details of the data are provided in Appendix C. The Euclidean distances between the expression profiles of the tumors in the original high-dimensional space are approximated

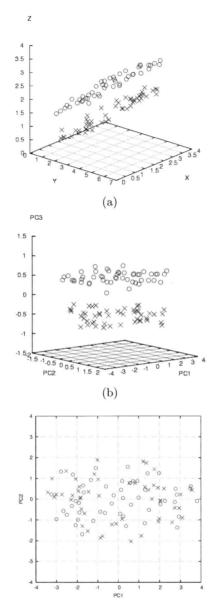

Fig. 9.2. (a) Three-dimensional scatterplot of hypothetical data arising from two subclasses denoted by × and o plotting symbols; (b) three-dimensional principal components representation of the data displayed in (a); (c) two-dimensional principal components representation of the data displayed in (a). Observe that the clear separation of the × and o subclasses has been lost in the dimension reduction.

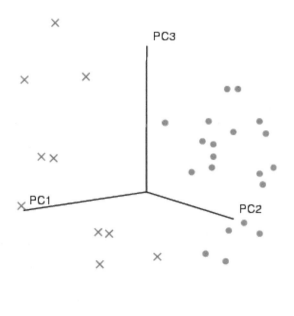

Fig. 9.3. Classical multidimensional scaling display of the gene expression profiles obtained for 31 melanoma tumors (Bittner et al. 2000). Distance metric used in original high-dimensional space was Euclidean distance. Orange filled circles correspond to 20 tumors belonging to an "interesting" cluster identified through hierarchical cluster analysis.

by the distances between the points in this three-dimensional display. The orange • plotting symbols denote tumors belonging to a cluster of interest that had been detected using cluster analysis algorithms (see Section 9.4), and the remaining tumors are plotted with blue × symbols. We discuss this plot further in later sections of this chapter.

Plotting symbol type, size, and color can be varied to enrich the amount of information conveyed in a multidimensional scaling display. For example, Figure 9.4 is a multidimensional scaling display that shows the degree of similarity among gene expression profiles (using cDNA microarrays with common reference design) obtained from fine needle aspirate (FNA) samples and excised tumors from a group of breast cancer patients. The data are described in detail in Assersohn et al. (2002). In this plot, small circles represent FNAs, large circles represent source tumor from which the FNAs were taken, and each color denotes a different patient. The conclusion to be drawn from this figure is that gene expression profiles from FNAs resemble the profile of their

MDS: Breast Tumor and FNA Samples

Color = Patient
Large circle = Tumor
Small circle = FNA

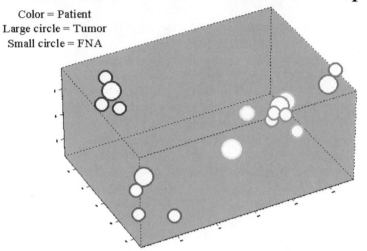

Fig. 9.4. Multidimensional scaling display of the gene expression profiles obtained for a collection of breast tumor specimens (large circles) and fine needle aspirate specimens (small circles). Data are from Assersohn et al. 2002. Different colors represent different patients. The distance metric used in the multidimensional scaling was one minus the Pearson correlation.

source tumor. In this group of patients, any minor differences that did exist between FNAs and their source tumor were generally small enough that the ability to distinguish between patients was not impaired. Because the distance metric used by Assersohn et al. (2002) to produce this multidimensional scaling display was one minus Pearson correlation instead of Euclidean distance, the display is slightly different than the principal components form of multidimensional scaling.

The examples we have presented thus far have involved graphical displays to examine relationships among specimens. In theory, multidimensional scaling displays could also be used to visualize genes, that is, one plotted point per gene. However, in practice the number of genes is usually very large and therefore it could be difficult to distinguish individual points and patterns in the display. It may be necessary to screen out genes, to use special colors or symbols for plotting the points, or to perform some preliminary data reduction through clustering of genes, for example, prior to producing the multidimensional scaling display. More is said in Section 9.4 about displays for visualizing gene clusters.

Here we have shown how the principal components can be useful for creating graphical displays. We note, however, that usually principal components will not be individually biologically interpretable because they are a weighted combination of a potentially large number of variables (combinations of expression measures for thousands of genes if examining classes of specimens).

9.3.2 Nonmetric Multidimensional Scaling

Rank-based multidimensional scaling methods have also been suggested. The method of nonmetric multidimensional scaling searches for a configuration of points in s-dimensional space for which the rankings of the interpoint distances in the original space are well preserved in the new space. Thus this method uses only the ranks of the interpoint distances, and discards the magnitudes. As in other rank-based statistical methods, non-metric multidimensional scaling will be less sensitive to extreme observations and noise in the data. However, this stability can come at the expense of decreased sensitivity for detecting true patterns in the data.

9.4 Clustering Algorithms

The goal of clustering methods is to form subgroups such that objects (specimens or genes) within a subgroup are more similar to one another than objects in different subgroups. A major distinction among types of clustering algorithms is the distinction between hierarchical methods and partitional methods (Jain et al. 1999), and examples of both types are discussed. Partitional methods aim to produce a single partition of the items, whereas hierarchical methods aim to find a nested series of partitions. K-means clustering and self-organizing maps are both partitional methods. Hierarchical agglomerative clustering and hierarchical divisive clustering are examples of hierarchical methods.

9.4.1 Hierarchical Clustering

Hierarchical clustering algorithms derive a nested series of partitions of data points. In the microarray context, each data point would consist either of the expression profile for a specimen or of the expression profile for a gene. Here we describe the methods in terms of clustering arrays, so data points are expression profiles for specimens. *Agglomerative hierarchical clustering* begins with each array as its own cluster and at each stage chooses the "best" merge of two arrays or two clusters of arrays until, in the end, all arrays are merged into a single cluster. *Divisive hierarchical clustering* proceeds in the opposite direction. It starts with all arrays in a single cluster and at each stage finds the best split. Divisive algorithms are less commonly used, perhaps because they are more computationally demanding. However, for dividing the set of arrays into relatively few large clusters, divisive methods may perform better than agglomerative clustering. We discuss here, however, only the more commonly used agglomerative hierarchical clustering. Eisen et al. (1998) were some of the first to apply agglomerative hierarchical clustering methods to microarray data.

9.4.1.1 Linkage Methods

The clustering procedure requires specification of both a similarity metric and a linkage. The similarity metric is defined for pairs of specimens. In hierarchical agglomerative clustering, the two most similar specimens are merged first, and then specimens or clusters of specimens are successively merged in order of greatest similarity. Although the similarity metric reflects distance between two individual specimens, additional specifications are required to define distance between two clusters. The specification of distance between clusters is determined by the *linkage method*. *Average linkage* uses the average distance between all pairs of items, one item from each cluster. *Complete linkage* uses the maximum distance between a member of one cluster and a member of the other cluster. *Single linkage* uses the minimum distance between a member of one cluster and a member of the other cluster.

Single linkage has a tendency to produce long "string-like" clusters (a phenomenon known as chaining). It is particularly sensitive to noise in the data and is regarded by many as an undesirable method. Yeung et al. (2001 b) found single-link hierarchical clustering to perform poorly for clustering genes for the gene expression microarray datasets they considered. Complete linkage tends to produce compact clusters of roughly equal size. Average linkage can be viewed as providing a compromise between the single linkage goal of wide separation between clusters and the complete linkage goal of compact clusters.

Both single linkage and complete linkage use only the rankings of the pairwise distances, and the clustering results obtained when using them will be invariant to any monotone transformation of the distance, for example, whether distances or squared distances are used. In contrast, average linkage does not have this invariance property, and some investigators find this an undesirable property. Gibbons and Roth (2002) examined the performance of several clustering methods on four publicly available yeast microarray datasets. In comparing the performance of single, complete, and average linkage hierarchical clustering for clustering genes, they found the performance of complete linkage to be substantially superior to both single and average linkage for recovering known functional classes of genes. For clustering specimens, we have found both complete and average linkage to be useful. We recommend against using single linkage for clustering either specimens or genes.

Numerous other linkage methods are available for use in hierarchical cluster analyses; see Gordon (1999) for an extensive discussion. We note here only two additional linkage methods besides those described above. One is that used by Eisen et al. (1998) and implemented in the "Cluster" software. Although referred to by Eisen as "average" linkage, it is not the same as the average linkage we describe above. Under Eisen's average linkage method, the distance between two clusters is computed as the distance between their centroids (cluster means). There are computational advantages to this method as the algorithm requires fewer calculations to determine best merges. However, it can lead to diffuse clusters that are not well separated.

Another linkage method that has enjoyed some popularity is Ward's method (Ward 1963). In Ward's method, the focus is on controlling the total sum of squared distances about the cluster centroids. At any stage, the optimal merge of clusters is the one that leads to the smallest possible increase in the total sum of squared distances about the cluster centroids. It is similar in spirit to complete linkage because both are aiming to produce "tight" clusters, but the two methods differ in the way they quantify "tight."

One disadvantage of hierarchical clustering procedures in general is that due to their sequential nature, they cannot recover from a bad merge (agglomerative algorithms) or split (divisive algorithms). Once a bad merge or split decision has been made, the algorithm must continue down that path. These bad decisions are most likely to occur when there is considerable noise in the data. Sometimes it is useful to apply a partitional clustering algorithm to the data such as K-means (see Section 9.4.2) as a final "clean-up" step after a hierarchical clustering has been applied. For example, if a hierarchical clustering is performed and it suggests five clusters are present in the data, one can perform K-means with five clusters using the cluster centroids from the hierarchical clustering as the initial centroids. Yeung et al. (2001b) found this clean-up step to yield improved clustering results in their investigations.

9.4.1.2 Dendrograms

The end result of a hierarchical clustering is a tree structure or *dendrogram*. Example dendrograms are presented in Figures 9.5(a) to (c). The dendrogram in Figure 9.5(a) resulted from hierarchical cluster analysis applied to log expression ratios from the melanoma data of Bittner et al. (2000) (31 tumors, 3613 genes as described for Figure 9.3). The distance metric used was one minus the Pearson correlation and average linkage was used. At the bottom of the tree, each of the original specimens constitutes its own cluster and, at the top of the tree, all specimens have been merged into a single cluster. The tree is "rooted" at the top. Mergers between two specimens, or between two clusters of specimens, are represented by horizontal lines connecting them in the dendrogram. The height of each horizontal line represents the distance between the two groups it merges, with greater heights representing greater distances. This is often not appreciated and sometimes software does not even preserve the height data which are very important to interpreting dendrograms.

Figures 9.6(a) and 9.6(b) were created from simulated data using hierarchical clustering with distance equal to one minus Pearson correlation and

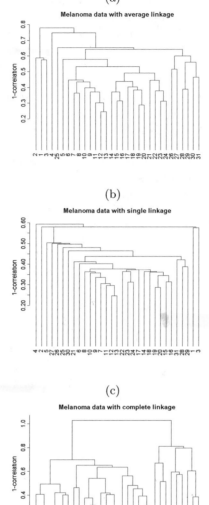

Fig. 9.5. Dendrograms resulting from hierarchical cluster analyses of gene expression profiles obtained for 31 melanoma tumors (Bittner et al. 2000). Distance metric used in all three dendrograms was one minus Pearson correlation. Linkage methods used were (a) average linkage, (b) single linkage, and (c) complete linkage.

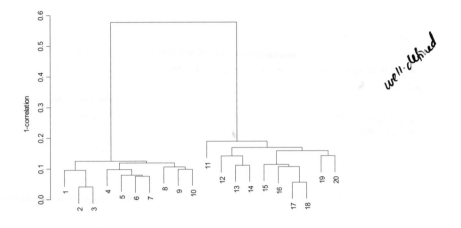

(a)

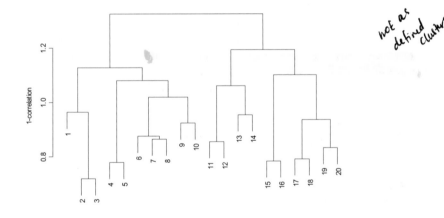

(b)

Fig. 9.6. Dendrograms created from two simulated datasets using average linkage hierarchical clustering with distance equal to one minus Pearson. For dendrogram (a), Gaussian data were simulated from two well-separated clusters. Data from random Gaussian noise were used to create dendrogram (b).

average linkage, and they illustrate the importance of labeling the vertical axis in a dendrogram. Both figures might convey the impression of two clusters. The data used for Figure 9.6(a) were Gaussian data generated from two well-separated clusters, and this figure does, in fact, exhibit two tight, well-separated clusters. The height at which the last merge occurs to complete the cluster of items 1 through 10 is approximately 0.12 (Pearson correlation = 0.88), and the cluster of items 11 through 20 is completed at a height of approximately 0.18 (Pearson correlation = 0.82). The distance between the two clusters is large; the height of their merge corresponds to a Pearson correlation of only 0.42. In contrast, all merges in Figure 9.6(b) occur at heights of 0.6 or greater (Pearson correlation less than 0.4). The data used to create Figure 9.6(b) were generated as random Gaussian noise; that is, there was no true clustering. (We labeled the arrays based on their resulting ordering in the dendrogram.) Any appearance of clusters in Figure 9.6(b) is due to chance.

Dendrograms in Figures 9.5(a),(b),(c) differ only in the linkage method used. It can be readily seen how changing the linkage method can substantially alter the results of the clustering, and therefore the appearance of the cluster dendrogram. For example, using complete linkage (Figure 9.5(c), tumors 1 to 4 appear to cluster with tumors 25 to 29 (albeit fairly late in the merging process). In contrast, using single linkage (Figure 9-5b) tumors 25 to 29 are dispersed throughout the dendrogram. It should be kept in mind, however, that the left-to-right ordering in the dendrogram is determined by an arbitrary rule that may differ between software implementations. The ordering rule used by the statistical software R is to place the tighter of the two just-merged clusters on the left. Tightness is determined by the linkage method, with singleton clusters being the tightest possible clusters. Eisen et al. (1998) suggest that when clustering genes by hierarchical clustering, one might determine left-to-right ordering based on the genes' average expression levels (across arrays) or chromosomal positions. The dendrograms in Figure 9.5 use the "tighter cluster to the left" rule. The fact that tumors 1 and 3 appear on the far left in the dendrogram of Figure 9.5(a) but on the far right in Figure 9.5(b) is of little significance. In both cases, those two tumors cluster first with each other and are some of the last to be clustered with any other tumors.

Figure 9.7 shows another hierarchical clustering dendrogram constructed from the same data, where in this case, median centering of the genes (see discussion at end of Section 9.2) has been performed prior to clustering. Note the difference between it and the dendrogram in Figure 9.5(a) that used the same similarity metric and linkage method. However, had we used Euclidean distance in the hierarchical clustering, the median centering of genes would not have affected the clustering results because the gene medians would "subtract out" in the Euclidean distance formula. All of the above dendrogram examples demonstrate the potential lack of stability of clustering results with regard to choice of cluster analysis method and data preprocessing. Some of this variation is to be expected because different clustering methods or data

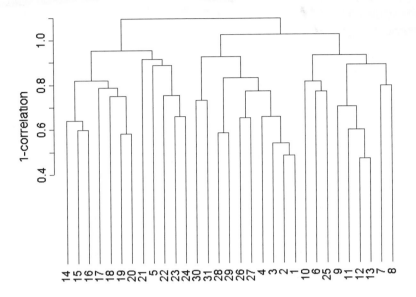

Fig. 9.7. Dendrogram resulting from average linkage hierarchical cluster analysis of gene expression profiles obtained for 31 melanoma tumors (Bittner et al. 2000). Prior to clustering, median centering of log ratios was performed within each gene. Distance metric was one minus Pearson correlation.

preprocessing methods may emphasize different aspects of the data, but some of the variation is pure instability resulting from noise in the data, the high-dimensionality of the data, and the relatively small number of arrays. Very strong clustering patterns (tight clusters and good separation between clusters, e.g., Figure 9.6(a) should be reasonably stable even when factors such as linkage method are varied, but different distance metrics or data centering methods might still have a very large impact on the clustering results. We recommend comparison of results obtained from application of multiple clustering methods in order to assess the level of this instability for any given dataset. Also, when trying to compare clustering patterns across different datasets, it should be kept in mind that the comparison could be completely confounded with the clustering algorithms used.

9.4.1.3 Color Image Plots

Another popular display method for hierarchical clustering results is a color image plot (also called a heatmap) that is a rectangular array of colored blocks, with the color of each block representing the expression level of one gene on one array (specimen). Typically, shades of red are used to represent degrees of increasing expression, and shades of green are used to represent degrees of decreasing expression. Each column of boxes represents a specimen, and each row of boxes corresponds to a gene. The columns are ordered according to how they are ordered in the hierarchical clustering dendrogram obtained from clustering specimens. In this case, the genes have also been subjected to a hierarchical clustering, and the rows are ordered according to how they were ordered in the dendrogram that resulted from the cluster analysis of genes. The end result is a color image plot with patches of red and green indicating combinations of genes and specimens that exhibit high or low expression. If one were clustering genes on the basis of time-series experiments and wanted to display the results in a color image plot, typically only the rows, and not the columns, would be ordered by hierarchical clustering.

Figure 9.8 presents an example color image plot for the same melanoma data used for the dendrograms just discussed. We have color-coded the blocks in this display by the values of the standardized log ratio, calculated by subtracting the mean log expression ratio for the array and dividing by the standard deviation. This puts the data on a scale that is more comparable to using a 1 - correlation distance metric. A red band of blocks (corresponding to a subset of genes) at the center top of the image plot seems to be one of the defining characteristics of the subgroup of tumors consisting of tumors 5 to 24 (with labels printed in orange). This is the "cluster of interest" reported by Bittner et al. (2000) except for the addition of tumor 5. See Section 9.5 for further assessment of this cluster. Other examples of color image plots are given in Eisen et al. (1998) and Alizadeh et al. (2000).

Care must be taken in interpreting the color-coding of the blocks when any standardization or centering of the data has been performed. For example, in Figure 9.8 expression measurements were standardized within each array, so the coloring of a particular block represents the number of standard deviations the expression measurement is away from the mean in that array, and these standardized values cannot be compared in an absolute sense between arrays. When median centering of genes has been performed, then the color-coding of a particular block should be interpreted as the amount of expression above or below the median for that gene. In this case, the values cannot be compared in an absolute sense across genes. The impact of median centering genes on the appearance of the image plot is that the red and green blocks are approximately balanced within each row (gene).

9.4.2 k-Means Clustering

The k-means method is a popular partitional clustering procedure. Given some specified number of clusters k, the goal is to segregate objects (specimens or genes) into k cohesive subgroups. (Note that the k in k-means should not be confused with K, the total number of genes.) A published example

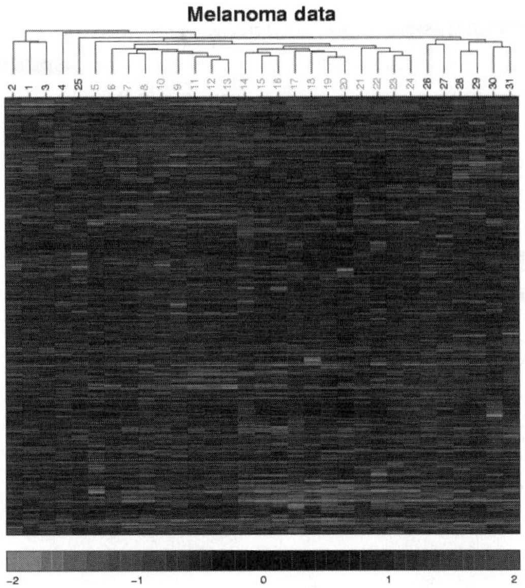

Fig. 9.8. Color image plot representing results of average linkage hierarchical cluster analysis of gene expression profiles obtained for 31 melanoma tumors (Bittner et al. 2000). Distance metric was one minus Pearson correlation. Tumors (columns) and genes (rows) are each ordered according to dendrogram order. At the top is the dendrogram resulting from the clustering of the tumors. Because the distance metric used for clustering was $1 -$ correlation, each block in this display has been color-coded by the value of its corresponding standardized log ratio (for each log expression ratio on each array, subtract the mean log expression ratio for the array and divide by the standard deviation for the array). Blocks colored most intense red represent the most highly over expressed genes, and blocks colored most intense green represent the genes with greatest degree of under expression. Black indicates genes whose expression is similar in the experimental and common reference samples. Note the red band of blocks (corresponding to a subset of genes) at the center top of the image plot. This appears to be one of the defining characteristics of the subgroup of tumors consisting of tumors 5 to 24 with tumor numbers printed in orange.

of its application to gene expression data is found in Aronow et al. (2001). The basic algorithm, as described by MacQueen (1967), begins with either an initial partition of the objects into k subgroups or an initial specification of k cluster centroids. These initial subgroups may represent a random partition of the dataset, or sometimes they are obtained from a preliminary hierarchical clustering or other clustering. Similarly, the initial centroids might be k randomly chosen points from the dataset or they might be centroids of clusters obtained from a preliminary hierarchical clustering dendrogram cut at some level. The algorithm proceeds by considering each object, one by one, and determining to which of the current cluster centroids the object is closest (usually as measured by Euclidean distance). The object is then "assigned" to that cluster. The centroid of the recipient cluster is updated to reflect its new member, and the centroid of the donor cluster (if there was an initial partitioning of objects) is updated to reflect the loss. The algorithm cycles through the data again, reallocating objects among the clusters and updating cluster centroids. The cycling ends when the entire list of objects has been presented without any more reallocations occurring. In practice, it is a good idea to run the algorithm multiple times using different initial partitions or centroids to assess sensitivity of the final results to the initial conditions. If different results are obtained, one might select the best partition by use of a criterion such as minimum sum of within-cluster distances.

A major advantage of nonhierarchical clustering methods such as k-means is computational feasibility. Unlike hierarchical methods, there is no need to compute or store all pairwise distances (or similarities) between objects. This makes it possible to cluster a larger number of objects in less time. In the context of microarray data, this is particularly important for clustering genes, which may number in the tens of thousands. Many computer implementations of hierarchical clustering cannot handle clustering of more than a few thousand genes. Disadvantages of k-means are that it does require specification of a number of clusters and an initial partitioning, and the final results can be very sensitive to these choices. Rahnenfuehrer (2002) compares several clustering methods on two microarray datasets with known clusters and finds that k-means (fixing the number of clusters) typically performed poorly when applied only a single time to a dataset. However, Rahnenfuehrer (2002) also considered a "best-of-10" k-means partition. This best-of-10 partition is obtained by applying the k-means algorithm 10 times to a single dataset using ten different randomly chosen sets of initial cluster centroids, and choosing the partition that minimizes the within-cluster sum of squares. This best-of-10 k-means partitioning method had very good performance on the two datasets considered by Rahnenfuehrer (2002). Another limitation of k-means is that less information is provided about the full structure of the data in the sense of similarity or dissimilarity among clusters. For example, in hierarchical clustering a dendrogram shows relationships among clusters. Graphical display of the k-means results such as a multidimensional scaling plot of the cluster centroids or of all of the data points with the clusters identified by color can be helpful.

Figure 9.9 is a parallel coordinates plot illustrating the relationship between the clusters derived using various hierarchical and k-means clustering methods applied to the melanoma data of Bittner et al. (2000). The first (lowest) level of circles represents the clusters derived by hierarchical clustering using the distance of one minus Pearson correlation and average linkage; the leftmost cluster is the 20-element cluster of tumors 5 to 24. The second level shows the clusters derived from hierarchical clustering with average linkage using Euclidean distance rather than one minus correlation distance. It can

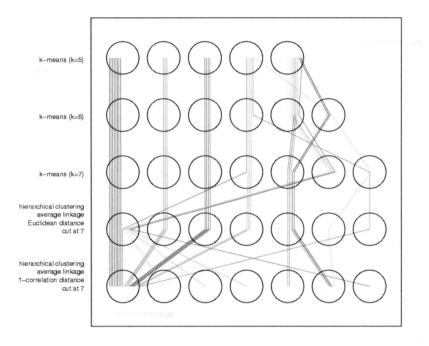

k−means (k=5)

k−means (k=6)

k−means (k=7)

hierarchical clustering
average linkage
Euclidean distance
cut at 7

hierarchical clustering
average linkage
1−correlation distance
cut at 7

Fig. 9.9. Parallel coordinates plot displaying results of multiple clustering methods applied to the melanoma data of Bittner et al. (2000). The first (lowest) level of circles represents the clusters derived by hierarchical clustering using distance of one minus Pearson correlation and average linkage; the left most cluster is the 20-element cluster of tumors 5 to 24 noted in Figure 9.3. The second level shows the clusters derived from hierarchical clustering with average linkage using Euclidean distance rather than one minus correlation distance. The third through fifth levels are based on k-means clustering with $k = 7$, 6, and 5, respectively. Each k-means result is the best obtained (smallest sum of squared distances from centroids) from among 10 separate k-means analyses, each using a different set of k initial cluster centroids selected randomly from the 31 tumor profiles.

be seen that changing the distance metric substantially alters the definitions of the clusters. Changing to the k-means clustering method ($k = 7$, 6, and 5 for levels 3, 4, and 5, respectively) defines yet another set of clusterings. For each of the k-means analyses ($k = 7$, 6, and 5), k initial cluster centroids were randomly selected (without replacement) from among the 31 tumor profiles. This random selection of k centroids was performed 10 times: the k-means clustering was derived for each initialization, and then the final k-means clustering result reported was the one of the 10 that produced the smallest sum of within-cluster sum of squared distances from centroids.

9.4.3 Self-Organizing Maps

Self-organizing maps (SOMs), developed and studied by Kohonen (1997), are
another clustering approach that has been used for the analysis of microarray
data. It can be viewed as a constrained version of the k-means algorithm in
which a relationship is maintained between cluster centroids. In this type of
analysis (assuming one is clustering arrays), a set of K-dimensional vectors
is mapped into a set of nodes in a lower-dimensional space. The nodes in
this lower-dimensional space have some imposed structure such as being arranged in a rectangular grid on a two-dimensional coordinate system. With
each node in the grid there is associated a K-dimensional vector, sometimes
called a *codebook value.* We denote the codebook value associated with the
jth node by c_j. Initially, codebook values are assigned at random to the grid
nodes, for example, by random selection from the data points or random generation on the range of the data. Then each vector in the dataset ("input
value") x is compared to the set of codebook vectors to determine to which
it is closest. That closest codebook value c_m and other codebook values corresponding to grid nodes within some neighborhood of the closest node (on
the two-dimensional grid) are moved toward the input value x by some multi-
plicative shrinkage factor $\alpha(t)$, called the *learning rate.* The procedure cycles
through the data, and as the iterations progress, both the learning rate and
the neighborhood size are decreased.

Symbolically, the iterated step in the SOM procedure can be described as
$c_j \leftarrow c_j + \alpha(t)(x - c_j)$ for all c_j associated with grid nodes in the neighborhood
$N_m(t)$ of node m for iterations $t = 1, 2, \ldots$. The procedure iterates through
the dataset multiple times until convergence of the codebook vectors is reached
or until $\alpha(t) = 0$. A popular choice for $\alpha(t)$ is a linear function that decreases
to zero by the time the maximum number of iterations is reached; a popular
choice for the neighborhood $N_m(t)$ is a "bubble" with radius that decreases
with the number of iterations. At the end, each input value is assigned to the
node having the codebook vector to which it is closest. In this way, clusters of
the original data vectors in K-dimensional space are formed and associated
with grid nodes in two-dimensional space. Neighboring grid nodes will have
associated with them codebook vectors that are more similar than codebook
vectors associated with nodes distant from each other on the two-dimensional
grid.

If one were to define the neighborhood size small enough that it never
contained any other grid nodes besides the one at its center, then codebook
vectors would be updated independently of each other. In this case, the SOM
procedure would reduce to an approximate k-means clustering with k equal
to the number of grid nodes.

There is obviously considerable subjectivity in the choice of grid size and
configuration, shrinkage function, and neighborhood size, and it is well known
that the final map can be sensitive to these choices. It is recommended that
multiple settings of these factors be considered to determine how much the

final results will vary. If the final map does not vary much, one can have greater confidence in the results.

Tamayo et al. (1999) fit a SOM to cluster genes in a time course experiment involving hematopoietic differentiation in HL-60 cells using the software GeneCluster available at `http://www-genome.wi.mit.edu/cancer/soft ware/software.html`. In this experiment, gene expression profiles were measured on cRNA samples prepared from HL-60 cell line cultures at 0, 0.5, 4, and 24 hours after exposure to the phorbol ester PMA. The array platform was the Affymetrix HU6000 expression array which contains probes to represent 6416 distinct human genes, of which 585 were used in the analysis because they showed sufficient variation across timepoints; see Appendix B for detailed information about the data. We conducted our own SOM analysis of these data, using the GeneSOM package (based on SOM_PAK-3.1 written in R, `http://www.stat.math.ethz.ch/CRAN/bin/windows/contrib/GeneSOM.zip`) to fit a 4×3 rectangular SOM with horizontal and vertical spacing of one unit. We used the same 585 genes as Tamayo, but we prefer to work on the log scale. We transformed the expression values to the log base 2 scale, and then each gene was standardized by subtracting its mean over the four time points and dividing by its standard deviation. (Tamayo et al. applied a similar standardization to each gene, but did not take log transformation.) We specified 10,000 iterations, an initial $\alpha = .1$ with linear decrease over the iterations, and a bubble neighborhood with initial radius $= 5$ and decreasing linearly to 1 over the iterations.

Figure 9.10 displays the results of the SOM fit. A multipanel figure of plots such as this is one of the most commonly employed display techniques for SOMs. For each node of the final SOM, an average time course (over the four timepoints) for the genes mapped to that node was computed. The arrangement of panels in the figure corresponds to the arrangement of nodes on the grid. The line plot displayed in each panel is the average time course for the genes mapped to that node, and the error bars at each timepoint indicate one standard deviation where the standard deviation is computed from the values recorded at that timepoint for those genes. For example, we see that the genes mapping to the nodes in the last row all exhibit expression levels that are relatively constant from baseline (time 0) through 4 hours, but then their expression levels decrease by 24 hours. We refer to the plot at each node as a *profile plot*. Similarity of the profile plots gives an indication of the closeness of the clusters. Although with four time points it is not too difficult for the eye to assess similarity of profile plots, for more complex profile plots over longer time courses, this assessment may be difficult. In these cases, it can be useful to cluster the codebook values using k-means or hierarchical clustering and visualize them using a multidimensional scaling display or dendrogram.

SOMs and k-means clustering share many of the same advantages and disadvantages. What we see as the major advantage of SOMs over hierarchical clustering is the computational feasibility when large numbers of objects (e.g., genes) are being clustered. For example, to cluster 5000 genes using hierar-

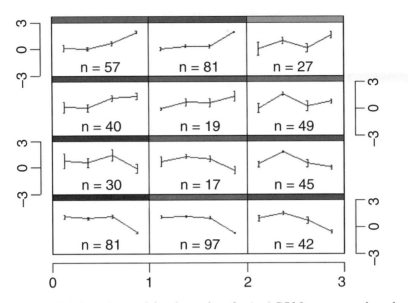

Fig. 9.10. Profile plots obtained for the nodes of a 4×3 SOM constructed to cluster genes in a time course experiment involving hematopoietic differentiation in HL-60 cells (Tamayo et al. 1999). Plotted values represent average log base 2 expression measurements, and error bars represent one standard deviation. The value of n designated for each node is the number of genes that were mapped to that node by the SOM analysis.

chical clustering would require calculation of millions of pairwise distances. Disadvantages are the sensitivity to grid configuration and other parameters such as neighborhood size, learning rate, and shrinkage function. Particularly, we have found cases where using too few grid nodes can lead to very poor performance, so we recommend erring on the side of too many grid nodes with the possibility of later combining or reducing the number of nodes. Also, as reported by Rahnenfuehrer (2002), sometimes the SOMs take a very long time (large number of iterations) to converge. Thus, although SOMs have been successfully applied to some microarray datasets, in general one should exercise caution in using them.

9.4.4 Other Clustering Procedures

There are many other clustering methods and it is beyond the scope of this book to cover even a modest fraction of them. However, we make note of just a few particularly interesting features of some other clustering procedures. The methods we have described up until this point are algorithmic rather than statistically based procedures. They all make assignments of each item to only one cluster rather than allowing for the possibility of membership in multiple clusters. Also, we have considered up to now only clustering arrays using similarity metrics based on all genes and clustering genes using similarity metrics based on all arrays. Briefly, we now discuss some alternative approaches.

One statistically based method of clustering involves the use of mixture models to determine clusters. Such approaches are often referred to as *model-based clustering*; see, for example, Banfield and Raftery (1992). Yeung et al. (2001a) discuss application of model-based clustering methods to microarray data. The Gaussian mixture model approach assumes that the data have arisen from a mixture of multivariate Gaussian distributions. For example, in clustering genes, the log expression vector for each gene (across the set of arrays) is assumed to have a multivariate Gaussian distribution characterized by a mean vector and a covariance matrix. Different clusters of genes are generated from different Gaussian distribution components. One can write the likelihood of the data as a function of the mean vectors and covariance matrices. Through maximum likelihood estimation, one can estimate the mean vector and covariance matrix of each of the component Gaussian distributions as well as the prevalences of the different components of the mixture. For each item considered in the clustering, one can estimate a probability that it came from any given cluster. These mixture model approaches are only possible to apply when the number of items (arrays or genes) being clustered exceeds the data dimension (number of genes if clustering arrays and number of arrays if clustering genes), and they are most likely to be successful when the number of items substantially exceeds the dimension. Consequently, this approach is most applicable to clustering genes. For clustering specimens, however, one would have to either restrict attention to a small number of genes, or use the first few (largest variance) principal components of the genes as the data, not individual genes. The R and Splus software packages both contain mixture model-based clustering routines.

Fuzzy clustering algorithms have the feature that they do not require each item to be assigned to only a single cluster. The output of a fuzzy clustering algorithm is a set of membership probabilities. Such algorithms might be particularly relevant for the clustering of genes. For example, we expect that some genes are involved in more than one pathway, and this could manifest itself as the gene belonging to more than one cluster. Jain et al. (1999) describe one basic version of a fuzzy clustering algorithm.

Several papers have proposed two-way clustering methods, that is, the simultaneous and nonindependent clustering of genes and specimens. The *plaid* model of Lazzeroni and Owen (2002) fits to gene-expression data sums of layers of two-way analysis of variance (ANOVA) models. In one of the ANOVA layers, a few subsets of genes may be showing increased or decreased expression in some subsets of specimens, whereas in another ANOVA layer, different subsets of genes may be exhibiting increased or decreased expression in different subsets of specimens. By adding together all of these layers, one can model complex situations such as genes potentially being involved in multiple pathways and influencing specimen profiles in multiple ways. As noted by its developers, a drawback to the complexity of the plaid model is that its fit can be sensitive to various options one specifies in the algorithm used to fit it, so considerable experimentation with fitting algorithms may be required to assure stable results. The *biclustering* method of Cheng and Church (2000) has similarities to the plaid models. It is an algorithm for searching for interesting gene-by-array subsets using ANOVA-type models, which is a slightly different goal than that of the plaid model which seeks to explain the expression data by summing up layered ANOVA models.

The *gene shaving* method was proposed by Hastie et al. (2000). It is designed to identify subsets of genes having high correlation in expression patterns that exhibit large variation across arrays. It can be effective in finding appropriate clusters when different subsets of specimens are driving different clusters of genes. Several authors have developed methods of finding subsets of genes that lead to interesting clustering of specimens (Ben-Dor et al. 2001; Xing and Karp 2001).

Sometimes investigators will use an informal approach to clustering genes on the basis of a subset of arrays or clustering arrays on the basis of a subset of genes. For example, from inspection of a color image plot produced using hierarchical clustering, it might be apparent that a particular subset of genes is mostly responsible for a cluster of arrays (specimens). It can be useful to refine the cluster by reclustering all arrays using only that subset of genes. In doing this, it is hoped that potential distortions in the clusters of arrays caused by including extraneous and possibly noisy data from other genes will be reduced. Applying class comparison procedures, such as *t*-tests or *F*-tests (Chapter 7) to compare gene expression profiles among the clusters is not valid, however, because the clusters were constructed based on the expression data rather than predefined based on phenotypes of the specimens. In the next section, we discuss more appropriate methods for evaluating clusters.

9.5 Assessing the Validity of Clusters

Clustering algorithms can find clusters even on random data. The clusters that are found by clustering algorithms will exhibit greater within-cluster homogeneity and more between-cluster separation than clusters formed by randomly partitioning the data because clustering algorithms can find spurious patterns in high-dimension random data. These features must be taken into account when attempting to objectively assess the validity of clustering results.

Assessing cluster validity is especially important when clustering specimens. We know that proteins are organized into pathways, that some genes are coregulated, and that some proteins are transcription factors involved in the transcriptional regulation of other genes. Consequently, the expression profiles of a large set of genes are expected to have structure. On the other hand, it is not clear a priori that the expression patterns of the specimens should have structure. If the specimens represent RNA extractions from disease tissue specimens of different patients, then the claim that there are real clusters is often a claim that the disease is not homogeneous and that different molecular subtypes have been discovered. This is a strong claim that requires more basis than simply that a clustering algorithm produced some clusters. In this section, we discuss some approaches for assessing clustering results. More extensive discussions can be found in Jain and Dubes (1988, Chapter 4) and Gordon (1999, Section 7.2).

Validation of a class predictor (Chapter 8) is far easier than validation of a classification obtained by a cluster analysis. For the former, there is known class information, and one can use cross-validation or bootstrap techniques on the data used to build the predictor, or one can test the predictor on a completely independent dataset for which class information is known. The difficulty in validating a cluster analysis-derived classification is that there is no gold standard classification against which the clustering results can be compared.

In lieu of a true gold standard classification, investigators sometimes will examine the relationship between the clustering results and external variables that have not been used in determining the clusters. For example, in studying cancer cell lines, one would likely know tissue type of origin of each of the cell lines, and it would be expected that a cluster analysis of the expression profiles of those cell lines should be able to recover that tissue type class structure. For clustering genes, it might be known that genes belong to certain functional classes and we might expect that at least some of that functional class structure would be picked up by the cluster analysis. Although it is not the goal to predict the values of those external variables or to rediscover the subgroups defined by those external variables, this exercise can lend some credibility to the clustering. However, the clustering will undoubtedly produce some clusters that are not readily explainable by the external information. This leaves one in a quandary as to whether the unexpected results are spurious or if they represent a truly novel and important finding. It is clear that additional approaches to cluster validity assessment are necessary. We focus on three main aspects of cluster validation: ① how to establish the presence versus complete absence of any clustering; ② how to find a good partition among many possible partitions of the data, and how to assess the reproducibility of a specific cluster.

9.5.1 Global Tests of Clustering

We use the term *global test* for clustering to refer to a test for the presence versus absence of clustering. To perform such global tests, one must have in mind some way of characterizing the degree of clustering in a set of points, and one must specify some null (no clustering) model to test. Some ways to characterize the degree of clustering include the distribution of pairwise interpoint distances or the distribution of nearest neighbor distances.

The concepts of pairwise and nearest neighbor distance distributions are illustrated in Figure 9-11. The leftmost plot in row (a) shows a scatter of points distributed completely at random over a circle with radius one. The scatterplot in row (b) shows a scatter of points generated from a bivariate normal distribution excluding points that fell outside the circle with radius one. Note that the scatterplots in rows (a) and (b) both could be regarded as showing a single cluster of points. However, a difference is that the cluster shown in the scatterplot in row (b) shows a higher density of points in the center of the circle with decreasing density moving outwards from the center, whereas the cluster in row (a) has a uniform density of points over the circle. The scatterplot in row (c) distinctly shows two clusters. The middle figure in each row is a histogram of nearest neighbor distances, and the last figure in each row is a histogram of pairwise distances. The differences in the scatterplots in rows (a) and (b) are reflected in both the nearest neighbor and pairwise distance histograms. The nearest neighbor histogram in row (b) shows an excess of small nearest neighbor distances (taller bar in smallest distance category) compared to the nearest neighbor distance histogram in row (a). This is picking up the higher density of points in the middle of cluster (b) compared to cluster (a). Also, the pairwise distance histogram in row (b) is more "pointed" and slightly skewed compared to the corresponding histogram in row (a). The most obvious difference in histograms is seen in comparing row (c) to row (a) or (b), in particular the bimodal pairwise distance histogram in row (c). Pairs of points with members drawn from the same cluster contribute most of the smaller pairwise interpoint distances comprising the left peak of the histogram, and pairs of points with members drawn from different clusters contribute most of the larger interpoint distances in the right peak of the histogram.

There are many plausible null models, and an inherent difficulty in conducting a test of no clustering is that the results can depend highly on the chosen null model. As previously stated, the scatterplots in both rows (a) and (b) of Figure 9.11 could be reasonably regarded as null models, yet if one were to test either one of them for clustering while specifying the other as the null model, the test would indicate significant departure from no clustering.

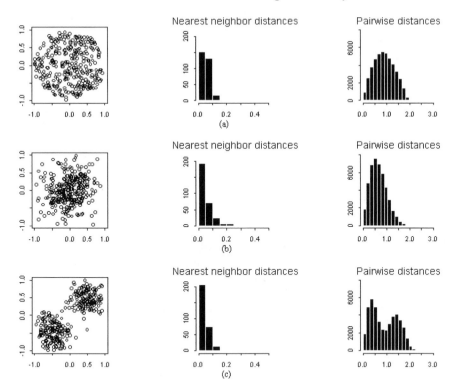

Fig. 9.11. Scatterplots (left column), nearest neighbor distance histograms (middle column), and pairwise distance histograms (right column) for three hypothetical datasets in two dimensions. In the top (row (a)) scatterplot, points were generated completely at random over a circle with radius one. Points in the middle (row (b)) scatterplot were generated from a bivariate normal distribution excluding points that fell outside the circle with radius one. In the bottom (row (c)) scatterplot, points were generated from two bivariate normal distributions with different means. The nearest neighbor distances are calculated by computing for each point in the dataset the distance from that point to the closest other point in the dataset. The pairwise distances are calculated by considering all possible pairings of points within the dataset, and then computing the interpoint distance within each pair.

Another type of null model that has been proposed (Harper 1978) is the one obtained by permuting the data, for example, permuting all of the expression values for different genes separately for each array. This approach is problematic when clustering specimens because it destroys the natural correlation among the genes, and this is not a null model of interest. Hence we do not recommend permutation methods for generating null data for assessing clustering of specimens.

The extremely high dimension of gene expression profile data makes it particularly challenging to specify an appropriate form for the null distribution in a global test. Typically, one must estimate from the data some parameters that define the null distribution. The higher the dimension, the more unknown parameters there are that must be assumed to have known values or must be estimated from the data. Errors in either the estimates or the assumed values can translate to huge errors in specification of the null distribution of points in the high-dimensional space, and this can cause extreme problems with the performance of statistical procedures. In our investigations we have found examples of global tests of clustering that perform very well in two- or three-dimensional space yet perform miserably in very high-dimensional space. This prompts a word of caution that one should not blindly assume that global tests of clustering that were developed for low-dimensional problems will automatically work well for high-dimensional gene expression data.

McShane et al. (2002) describe a global test of clustering for testing for the presence of any clustering in a collection of specimens. They base their test on the first three principal components (multidimensional scaling representation) for the specimens, and then they test for clustering in this three-dimensional space. This avoids the high-dimensionality problems described above, and they found their test to have good properties in simulation studies based on several high-dimensional expression datasets. In our experience many important clustering patterns can be detected using just the first three principal components. McShane et al. (2002) argue that a null distribution of a single trivariate normal distribution is reasonable because the principal components are weighted combinations of large numbers of variables, and therefore their distribution will tend to look normal; the mean and variance of that null distribution is estimated from the data. The McShane et al. (2002) quantification of clustering is based on the distribution of nearest neighbor distances. Applying their global test to the melanoma data of Bittner et al. (2000), described in Section 9.4.1.2, resulted in a p-value 0.01 for the test of no clustering. Hence they concluded that there was significant evidence for clustering of the expression profiles of the melanoma tumors.

9.5.2 Estimating the Number of Clusters

Once it is established that there does exist clustering in the data, a next logical step is to determine a good partition of the data or how many clusters there are in the data. There is an extensive literature on determining the number of clusters in multivariate data. A comprehensive review of 30 different procedures is given by Milligan and Cooper (1985). Many of these procedures are based on measures of cohesiveness within clusters versus separation between clusters, measures of the predictive power of the clustering (as described below), or on data perturbation methods in which stability of a partition in the presence of jittering (added random noise) is assessed. We discuss, in turn, several of these approaches that have been applied to microarray data.

Yeung et al. (2001b) propose use of a figure-of-merit (FOM)   criterion for estimating the predictive power of a clustering and choosing an optimal number of clusters. Their procedure is performed by removing one array at a time from the dataset, clustering the genes into k clusters based on the remaining data, and then assessing how well those k gene cluster means can predict the gene expression in the left-out array. Each array is left out, in turn, and the predictive measure is averaged over the arrays to produce the FOM. This procedure is repeated for different values of k and the FOM is then plotted against the number of clusters k. The number of clusters at which it reaches a minimum is taken to be the estimate of the optimal number of clusters. Their particular interest was in clustering genes and they relied on the independence of the arrays for justification of their leave-one-out approach. It is not clear that their method should be applied to clustering specimens, as it is not reasonable to assume that genes are independent.

Tibshirani et al. (2001) proposed the *GAP statistic* for estimating the number of clusters in multivariate data. It is based on a statistic that is equal to a pooled within-cluster sum of squares around the cluster means. The value of the GAP statistic observed for the data is compared to the sampling distribution expected under a null distribution described in their paper to determine the number of clusters that produces a partition most significantly different from that expected under the null distribution. In their paper, they applied it to a microarray data example in which they were trying to find the optimal number of clusters of arrays, although their reported simulation studies evaluated situations only up to dimension 10. Unfortunately, the GAP statistic appears to break down in high-dimensional microarray settings. Dudoit and Fridlyand (2002) reported that it overestimates the number of clusters in microarray data. Our own simulation studies have indicated that it will frequently erroneously find clusters in high-dimensional data that were generated from a single unimodal distribution. Hence it should not be used for determination of the number of clusters in microarray data.

Golub et al. (1999) suggested a cross-validation method for assessing clustering results that involves building a predictor for the observed clusters and assessing whether new expression profiles can be unambiguously assigned to specific clusters. Without an independent dataset, however, the method is problematic because the same data is used to build the clusters, develop the predictor, and evaluate classification error. The method could potentially be applied in the context of leave-one-out cross-validation (see Section 8.4.2).

Two cautions are in order regarding application of procedures for estimating the number of clusters to microarray data. The first is that procedures that work well in lower dimensions do not necessarily work well in the high-dimensional setting of microarrays. The failure of the GAP statistic for microarray data is a good example of this. In addition, there is a temptation to use these procedures that are designed for estimating the number of clusters as global tests (i.e., to demonstrate that the best estimate of the number of clusters is greater than one versus only one). Many of these procedures were not designed to differentiate between no clustering versus some number of clusters more than one. It should not be assumed without further investigation that they will perform well as global tests of clustering, because they may not have been designed to control the probability of falsely estimating that the number of clusters is greater than one in situations in which there are no clusters in the data. Moreover, some of the tests cannot even be calculated for the case of one cluster.

9.5.3 Assessing Reproduciblity of Individual Clusters

McShane et al. (2002) argue that it may be more useful to think in terms of assessing reproducibility of individual clusters rather than trying to find an "optimal number" of clusters. For example, it could be that a dataset contains only a few very strong clusters in the midst of "noise" points that don't fall neatly into clusters. Because a cluster algorithm will have to deal somehow with those noise points, it likely will either lump them in with one or more of the tight clusters (thus weakening those clusters) or will form additional small, not very reproducible clusters to encompass them. Consequently, either the average strength (over all clusters) of the resulting clusters or the number of clusters could be misleading. Both the methods of McShane et al. (2002) and those of Kerr and Churchill (2001 b) focus more heavily on assessing validity of individual clusters rather than estimating the number of clusters.

McShane et al. (2002) and Kerr and Churchill (2001 b) each considered data perturbation methods for assessing clustering results. The general approach of data perturbation to assess clustering stability is a technique that has been used by others in different settings (Rand, 1971; Gnanadesikan et al. 1977; Fowlkes and Mallows 1983).

Two cluster reproducibility measures were proposed by McShane et al. (2002) for assessing the meaningfulness of clusters of specimens. The idea is to assess the stability of the observed specimen clusters in the background of experimental noise. "New data" are simulated by adding artificial experimental error in the form of Gaussian noise to the existing log expression measurements. An appropriate variance to use in generating this Gaussian experimental error can be estimated on a gene-specific basis if replicate arrays are available. Otherwise, an approximate variance can be generated in the following way. For each gene, the variance across arrays of the expression measurements is calculated. If it is felt that the majority of genes will not be differentially expressed across arrays, then the median (50th percentile) of the observed distribution of variances can be taken as the experimental variance estimate. The median should be robust to contamination by modest numbers of large standard deviation estimates that reflect true tumor-to-tumor differences rather than experimental noise. A lower percentile such as the 10th or 25th may be a good choice if larger numbers of differentially expressed genes are expected.

The new "perturbed" data are then re-clustered and the results are compared to the original clustering results by calculating two different comparison measures. The first measure they call the robustness (R) index, and the second measure they call the discrepancy (D) index. The perturbation-clustering cycle is repeated numerous times to estimate the stability of the original clustering to data perturbations. Considering a particular number of clusters (for example, cutting the dendrogram from a hierarchical clustering at a particular level for both the original and perturbed data clusterings), the R-index measures the proportion of pairs of specimens within a cluster for which the members of the pair remain together in the re-clustered perturbed data. The D-index measures the number of discrepancies (additions or omissions) comparing an original cluster to a best-matching cluster in the reclustered perturbed data.

More specifically, the R-index is calculated as follows. Each of the original data dendrogram and the perturbed data dendrogram are cut to form k clusters. If a cluster i of the original data contains n_i specimens, it can be viewed as containing $m_i = n_i(n_i - 1)/2$ pairs of specimens. If the clusters are robust, then members of a pair should fall in the same cluster in the re-clustered data. Let c_i denote the number of these m_i pairs with members falling in the same cluster in the reclustered perturbed data. Then $r_i = c_i/m_i$ is a measure of the robustness of the ith cluster in the original dataset. For singletons, r_i is defined as the proportion of re-clusterings in which the specimen remains a singleton. An overall measure for the set of k clusters is $R = (c_1 + c_2 + \cdots + c_k)/(m_1 + m_2 + \cdots + m_k)$. Note that this overall measure is a weighted average of the cluster-specific measures, weighted by cluster size. In computing the overall measure, singleton clusters in the original data are excluded. The robustness indices are averaged over a large number of cycles of perturbations and re-clusterings. We suggest the benchmarks of an R-index of at least 0.9 for strong reproducibility of an individual cluster, or at least 0.8 for moderate reproducibility.

The D-index is computed somewhat differently. For each cluster of the original data, determine the cluster of the perturbed data that is the "best match," defined as the one having the greatest number of elements in common with the original cluster. (Ties are broken by choosing the match with the least number of added elements.) The discrepancy can be subdivided into one of two types; either specimens in the original cluster that are not in the best match perturbed cluster (omissions), or elements in the best match cluster that were not in the original cluster (additions). It can be helpful to keep track of these two types separately, and this is one potential advantage of the D-index compared to the R-index. An overall measure of discrepancy is the summation of cluster-specific discrepancy indices. These indices can also be averaged over a large number of cycles of perturbations and re-clusterings. In computing the discrepancy index, it is useful to consider cuts of the perturbed data tree with similar, in addition to identical, numbers of clusters as in the original data, and to report the D-index as the minimum over the several cuts considered.

Table 9.2. Cluster-Specific Reproducibility Measures for the Melanoma Data[a]

Cut at 7 Clusters		Overall: R-index = 0.992, D-index = 1.904[b]		
Cluster	Tumor members	Robustness[c]	Omissions	Additions
1	1, 3	.050	.928	.000
2	2	.960	.000	.000
3	4	1.00	.000	.000
4	5–24	1.00	.004	.008
5	25	.999	.000	.001
6	26–27	.954	.046	.465
7	28–31	.920	.209	.243

Cut at 8 Custers		Overall: R-index = 0.991, D-index = 17.334[b]		
Cluster	Tumor members	Robustness[c]	Omissions	Additions
1	1, 3	.000	.959	.000
2	2	1.00	.000	.000
3	4	1.00	.000	.000
4	5	.000	.000	14.853
5	6–24	1.00	.021	.782
6	25	.996	.000	.001
7	26–27	.920	.123	.142
8	28–31	.916	.386	.067

[a] A hierarchical agglomerative clustering algorithm using average linkage and distance metric equal to one minus the Pearson correlation was applied; 1000 simulated perturbed datasets were generated using a noise SD = .52.
[b] The D-index, omissions, and additions computed here allow searching over numbers of clusters in the perturbed data ranging from two less to two more than the number of clusters considered in the original data.
[c] The reported robustness measure for a singleton cluster is the proportion of perturbed data clusterings for which it remained a singleton in the perturbed data clustering.

Table 9.2 presents cluster-specific reproducibility measures for clusters formed at cuts of 7 and 8 clusters when hierarchical clustering with distance = 1−correlation and average linkage was applied to the melanoma data described in Section 9.3 and Appendix B. The estimated experimental noise standard deviation (square root of median estimated variance) estimate was 0.52 (log base 2 scale) for these data. Of particular interest to Bittner et al. (2000) was the 19-member cluster containing tumors 6 to 24 as shown in the central portion of the dendrogram in Figure 9.5(a). That group of 19 tumors occurs as a stand alone cluster at cuts of 8, 9, and 10 clusters. Cutting the tree at 8 clusters, it is evident from the reproducibility measures that, on average, there is an addition of about one member to the collection 6 to 24. The observation of a large average number of additions (14) to the singleton cluster containing tumor 5, along with inspection of several of the perturbed data trees (not shown), reveals that tumor 5 is frequently merged with tumors 6 to 24 when cutting to obtain 8 clusters. Going back to cutting the tree at 7 clusters, we see that the cluster with elements 5 to 24 (composed of Bittner et al.'s major cluster and one additional tumor) is highly reproducible. Thus there appears to be strong evidence for reproducibility of a large cluster containing tumors 5 to 24. These results support Bittner et al.'s identification of subsets of melanoma within the dataset with the minor refinement of tumor 5 being included with the major cluster of noninvasive melanomas.

Kerr and Churchill (2001 b) used data perturbation methods to assess the validity of select gene clusters in yeast microarray data for which they had predefined prototype profiles. These profiles (clusters) of interest were based on seven prespecified temporal patterns of induced transcription. To each profile of interest they assigned a hand-selected set of a few genes that they determined fit the profile, and then they calculated a prototype for that profile as the average of those initial genes selected for that profile. Their goal was to determine which of some candidate new genes showed strong evidence for inclusion in those clusters. They generated experimental noise for the perturbations by calculating residuals from an analysis of variance model fit to intensity measurements and bootstrapping from the empirical distribution of those residuals. For each gene, they recorded for the perturbed datasets the proportion of times that gene's profile best matched the prototype profiles of each of the prespecified gene clusters, where the best match was defined as the prototype profile having the highest correlation with that gene's profile. Although their primary goals were somewhat different from those of the McShane et al. (2002) methods which were used in the Bittner et al. (2000) study, they alluded to the idea of using an index equivalent to McShane et al.'s (2002) overall R-index in cases where there are no prespecified clusters or prototype profiles. Their methods required replicate profile measurements from at least some specimens, and the type of replicates available must be consistent with the totality of sources of experimental error that one wishes to account for in the reproducibility assessment. In our experience with microarray data, when replicates are available they often incorporate only some sources of the total experimental variation, for example, hybridization of a single sample to the multiple arrays, but not replication at the level of resampling a tumor or reisolating mRNA. In settings where appropriate replicates are available, the bootstrap resampling method for generating perturbation errors is an idea worthy of consideration, although it can be quite computationally intensive. If duplicate arrays of independent RNA extractions from the same tissue sample are available for a sufficient number of patients, then examining the extent to which duplicate samples appear in the same cluster can be potentially more informative than the statistical measures of cluster reproducibility.

A

Basic Biology of Gene Expression

A.1 Introduction

This appendix contains a brief introduction to the biology of gene expression for readers with little or no biological background. For more complete information with excellent illustrations, the reader can see references such as Watson et al. (1987).

The cell is considered the basic unit of life. A defining characteristic of life is reproduction. Single-celled organisms reproduce by cell duplication. Multicellular organisms start with a single cell and develop by the programmed division of cells.

Most of the important functions performed in cells involve proteins. A protein can be represented as a linear sequence of amino acids joined by peptide bonds (Figure A.1). Each amino acid consists of a central carbon atom to which three chemical entities are joined: the amine (NH_2) group, the carboxyl (COOH) group, and the side chain (R). There are 20 commonly occurring types of side chains and thus 20 amino acids (Figure A.2). The peptide bond connecting amino acids joins the nitrogen atom at the amino end of one amino acid to the carbon atom at the carboxyl end of the adjacent amino acid. Typical proteins contain between 100 to 1000 amino acids.

Although the chemical composition of a protein may be described by specifying the linear sequence of amino acids, the functional aspects of a protein are determined by the three-dimensional structure that the protein takes when placed in an aqueous solution. It was demonstrated by Sela et al. (1957) that the amino acid sequence determines the structural conformation of the protein but, to date, three-dimensional structure cannot be effectively predicted based on amino acid sequence.

Proteins do not self-assemble. They are assembled based on information contained in DNA. Messenger RNA (mRNA) acts as an intermediate: mRNA is synthesized using DNA as a template and is then used for translation into protein. All RNA molecules consist of a sequence of nucleotides (Figure A.3). There are four types of nucleotides in RNA: adenine (A), cytosine (C), gua-

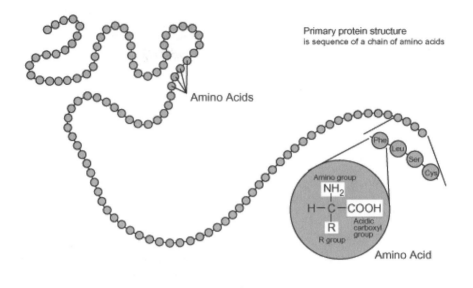

Fig. A.1.

nine (G), and uracil (U). Cytosine and uracil are single ring structures called pyrimidines whereas adenine and guanine are double ring structures called purines. Each nucleotide building block has a sugar-phosphate group attached to a specific side group. The sugar-phosphate units link together to form a backbone.

Each mRNA molecule is created by a multi-step process starting with a transcription using genomic DNA as a template for the construction of an RNA molecule. DNA is a polymer of nucleotides, in many ways similar to RNA. A DNA molecule consists of a string of nucleotides joined by a deoxyribose sugar backbone, rather than a ribose sugar backbone as in RNA. Whereas the nucleotides appearing in RNA are A, C, G, and U, in DNA thymine (T) replaces uracil (U). The bonds joining the nucleotides in DNA are directional, with what are referred to as a 5′ end and a 3′ end.

Although RNA and DNA share many features, there are also major differences. Whereas RNA molecules are short, the entire human genome consists of only 23 pairs of huge DNA molecules. These DNA molecules are packaged in the 23 pairs of chromosomes. Each of the DNA molecules consists of two strands of polynucleotides, wound around each other in a helical structure (Figure A.3). The structure is stabilized by chemical bonds between pairs of complementary bases on the two strands. The adenines (A) bind with thymines (T) and the guanines (G) bond with the cytosines (C) by hydrogen bonds. This complementarity of bases is a crucial feature of DNA; it is the basis of both cell reproduction and gene expression.

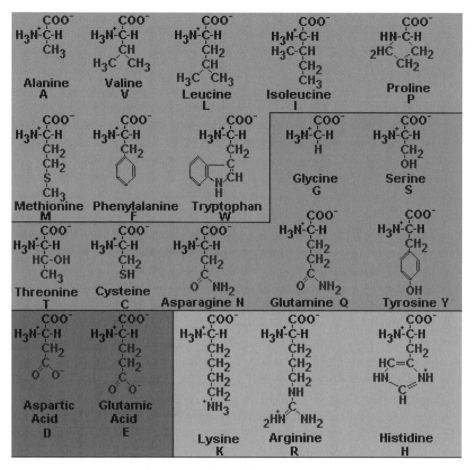

Fig. A.2.

In gene expression, the two strands of a DNA molecule separate and a molecule of RNA is synthesized using a segment of one of the DNA strands as a template (Figure A.4). The transcription occurs in the direction from the 5′ to 3′ end of the DNA segment. The DNA segment used for synthesis corresponds roughly to a single gene. The RNA molecule synthesized is complementary to the DNA sequence in the gene. That is, an adenine nucleotide in the DNA strand results in the synthesis of a uracil nucleotide in the growing RNA strand, a cytosine in the DNA strand results in the synthesis of a guanine in the RNA strand, a guanine in the DNA strand results in the synthesis of a cytosine in the RNA strand, and a thymine in the DNA strand results in the synthesis of an adenine in the growing RNA strand.

The transcription of the DNA into a messenger RNA molecule begins with the binding of the enzyme RNA polymerase to the DNA in the promoter region upstream of the 5′ start of the gene. That region contains control sequences

Ribonucleic acid(RNA)

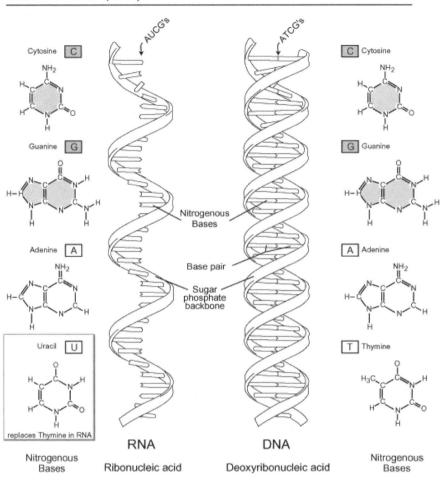

Fig. A.3.

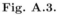

that are binding sites for proteins, called transcription factors, that influence the binding of RNA polymerase. Hence these sequences control the conditions under which the gene will be transcribed. The transcribed RNA molecule contains a sequence complementary to the DNA strand that served as the template. In multi-cell organisms, the created RNA molecule also contains a long string of adenines (As) added at the end of the segment, the so-called poly-A tail.

Genes of higher organisms are organized with segments of protein coding regions interspersed among longer segments of noncoding regions. The former

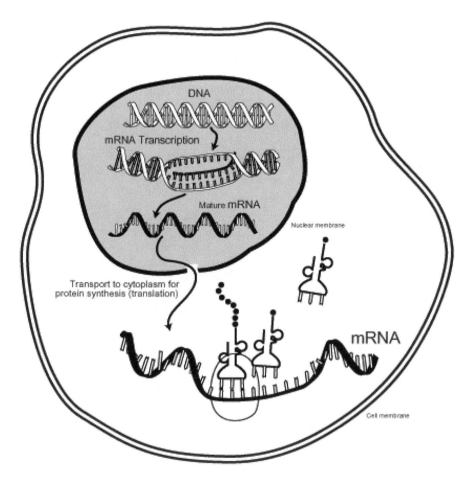

Fig. A.4.

are called exons and the latter introns. The intronic regions are excised from the mRNA molecule and the resulting exonic regions are spliced together. The poly-A tail is retained. Although the splicing process is not well understood, it is known that different kinds of mRNA transcripts, and consequently different protein variants, are obtained from transcription of the same gene by alternative splicings of the primary transcripts.

A spliced mature mRNA molecule exits the nucleus and is transported to a ribosome in the cytoplasm where it directs the synthesis of a molecule of protein. The ribosomes are complex structures consisting largely of RNA molecules of a different type called ribosomal RNA. Most of the RNA content of a cell is ribosomal RNA. At the ribosome, the mRNA molecule directs the synthesis of a protein molecule via the genetic code (Figure A.5). Triplets

FIRST BASE	SECOND BASE: U	SECOND BASE: C	SECOND BASE: A	SECOND BASE: G	THIRD BASE
U	UUU Phe	UCU Ser	UAU Tyr	UGU Cys	U
U	UUC Phe	UCC Ser	UAC Tyr	UGC Cys	C
U	UUA Leu	UCA Ser	UAA Stop	UGA Stop	A
U	UUG Leu	UCG Ser	UAG Stop	UGG Trp	G
C	CUU Leu	CCU Pro	CAU His	CGU Arg	U
C	CUC Leu	CCC Pro	CAC His	CGC Arg	C
C	CUA Leu	CCA Pro	CAA Gln	CGA Arg	A
C	CUG Leu	CCG Pro	CAG Gln	CGG Arg	G
A	AUU Ile	ACU Thr	AAU Asn	AGU Ser	U
A	AUC Ile	ACC Thr	AAC Asn	AGC Ser	C
A	AUA Ile	ACA Thr	AAA Lys	AGA Arg	A
A	AUG Met	ACG Thr	AAG Lys	AGG Arg	G
G	GUU Val	GCU Ala	GAU Asp	GGU Gly	U
G	GUC Val	GCC Ala	GAC Asp	GGC Gly	C
G	GUA Val	GCA Ala	GAA Glu	GGA Gly	A
G	GUG Val	GCG Ala	GAG Glu	GGG Gly	G

Fig. A.5.

of contiguous nucleotides, called *codons*, correspond to specific amino acids. Because there are only 20 naturally occurring amino acids, and there are 4^3 or 64 possible codons, the genetic code is redundant. In many cases the amino acid is determined by the first two nucleotides of the codon. Nevertheless, the translation process is based strictly upon the decoding of triplet codons without gaps between codons in the mRNA sequence.

The process of converting an mRNA molecule to a protein is called *translation*. Translation of mRNA involves a third type of RNA molecule, called transfer RNA (tRNA). A unique tRNA molecule exists for each possible codon. A tRNA molecule has an *anticodon* at one end, which binds to its corresponding codon. At the other end, the tRNA molecule has the corresponding amino acid. The anticodons of tRNA molecules bind to the corresponding codons of the mRNA molecule and thereby bring the correct sequence of amino acids together; peptide bonds form between adjacent amino acids.

A correspondence exists between protein molecules and mature mRNA molecules. Mature mRNA molecules are often called mRNA transcripts, because they are synthesized by transcription of DNA. Each synthesized molecule of protein requires and consumes one transcript, therefore the rate of synthesis of a protein can be estimated by quantifying the abundance of corresponding transcripts. The relationship between the rate of protein synthesis and abundance of transcripts of the corresponding type is not exact, however, because some transcripts are degraded before participating in protein translation, and the rate of degradation varies for different genes. Nevertheless, DNA microarrays are assays for measuring the abundance of mRNA transcripts corresponding to thousands of different genes in a collection of cells.

For the most part, all cells of a multicellular organism contain the same DNA. The cells differ from each other in function, and the functions of individual cells change over time based on external conditions. These functional differences are determined by differences in the abundance of the various types of proteins. Hence, by quantifying the abundance of mRNA transcripts in collections of cells from different tissues and under different conditions, one can gain insight into the biological mechanisms that mediate those differences.

B

Description of Gene Expression Datasets Used as Examples

B.1 Introduction

This appendix describes the datasets used as examples in this book. We have made versions of these datasets available on our Web site http://linus.nci. nih.gov/BRB-ArrayTools.html. These datasets are formatted for ease of importation into BRB-ArrayTools, and the names and formats of the files are described in Appendix C. Readers wishing to analyze these datasets using other software can either use the version described in Appendix C or can obtain the primary data directly from the Web sites of the original investigators who generated the data, as described below.

B.2 Bittner Melanoma Data

The data of Bittner et al. (2000) consist of gene expression profiles obtained on a collection of 38 samples, comprised of 31 melanoma tumors and 7 controls. The data were downloaded from http://research.nhgri.nih. gov/microarray/Melanoma_Supplement/Files/gene_list-Cutaneous_ Melanoma.xls. The array platform was a spotted cDNA array containing probes from 8150 cDNAs (representing 6971 unique genes). A common reference design was used for this series of experiments. The common reference sample was a pool of RNA from a nontumorigenic revertant of a melanoma cell line. Each test sample was labeled with Cy5 and the reference sample was labeled with Cy3. Thus a spot that shows up red in an image display corresponds to a large ratio (i.e., a gene that is more highly expressed in the test sample than the reference sample).

For the analyses presented in this book, the data from the seven control specimens were excluded, and only measurements from the 3613 genes that were considered "strongly detected" were used. Strongly detected spots were defined by Bittner et al. (2000) as those having an average mean intensity above the background of the least intense signal (Cy3 or Cy5) across all experiments greater than 2000, and an average spot size across all experiments greater than 30 pixels. An indicator variable is provided in the dataset to identify strongly detected spots. Only the ratios were made available on Bittner's Web site and they had already been normalized using image processing software. An additional processing step was to replace ratios greater than 50 by 50, and ratios less than 0.02 by 0.02. We have taken logarithms to the base 2 in the data we make available.

B.3 Luo Prostate Data

The data of Luo et al. (2001) consist of gene expression profiles obtained on a collection of 25 prostate tissue samples, comprised of 16 prostate cancers and 9 benign prostatic hyperplasia (BPH) specimens. The data were downloaded from http://research.nhgri.nih.gov/microarray/Prostate_Supplement/Images/6500GeneListw=CRs&QSs.xls. The array platform was a spotted cDNA array containing probes from 6500 human cDNAs (representing 6112 unique genes). A common reference design was used for this series of experiments. The common reference sample was a pool of RNA derived from two benign prostatic hyperplasia specimens. Each test sample was labeled with Cy3 and the reference sample was labeled with Cy5. Thus a spot that shows up green in an image display corresponds to a large ratio and a gene that is more highly expressed in the test sample than the reference sample. Only the ratios were made available by Luo et al. and they had already been normalized using image processing software. Quality scores taking values in the range zero to one were provided for each ratio measurement. A quality score of zero indicates that the ratio is unreliable and should not be used; positive quality scores increasing toward the highest quality level of one indicate increasing levels of measurement quality. Although the exact calculation method for the quality score is not reported, it is said to be a composite index that reflects the idea that unreliable datapoints frequently result from weak target intensity, high local background, small target area, and inconsistent target intensity within a given target. A subsequent report from the same group discusses their method for calculating quality scores (Chen et al. 2002). For the analyses presented in this book, only ratios with quality scores greater than zero are used. We have taken logarithms to the base 2 of the ratios in the file we provide.

B.4 Perou Breast Data

The data of Perou et al. (2000) include gene expression profiles obtained on a collection of 65 human breast tissue samples from 42 different individuals (36 infiltrating ductal carcinomas, 2 lobular carcinomas, 1 ductal carcinoma in situ, 1 fibroadenoma, and 3 normal breast samples). For the analyses presented in this book, the only expression profile data used were those from 20 breast cancer patients for whom specimens were available both before and after a 16-week course of doxorubicin chemotherapy. The microarray analyses generated two gene expression profiles for each of these 20 patients, one before and one after chemotherapy. The primary data were downloaded from `http://genome-www.stanford.edu/breast_cancer/molecularportraits/download.shtml`. The array platform was a spotted cDNA array. A common reference design was used for this series of experiments. The common reference sample was a pool of RNA isolated from 11 different cultured cell lines, and it was labeled with Cy3. Each test sample was labeled with Cy5. Thus a spot that shows up red in an image display corresponds to a large ratio and a gene that is more highly expressed in the test sample than the reference sample. Of the 9216 spots for which data were available, 185 were labeled as "EMPTY" and were flagged to be excluded from analysis. Data from spots flagged for quality reasons and not used by the original investigators were also excluded from the analyses in this book. In each channel the signal for a spot was calculated as foreground intensity minus background. Spots for which the signal was less than 100 in both channels were not used. If the signal was less than 100 in only one channel, the spot was used with the signal set in that channel to 100. The expression ratio was formed as channel 2 divided by the channel 1 signal. Ratios were median-normalized within each array by dividing the ratios by the median of the ratios for that array.

B.5 Tamayo HL-60 Data

The HL-60 data analyzed in Tamayo et al. (1999) consist of gene expression profiles obtained from a time-series experiment conducted on a cell line model of human hematopoietic differentiation. The myeloid leukemia cell line HL-60 undergoes macrophage differentiation when treated with the phorbol ester PMA. Antisense cRNA was prepared from the cells harvested at 0, 0.5, 4, and 24 hours after administration of PMA. The array platform was the Affymetrix HU6000 expression array containing probe sets for 6416 distinct human genes. Expression data were reported for 7229 probe sets because some genes were represented by more than one probe set, and there were a few additional probe sets to detect spiked controls. The data were downloaded from `http://www.genome.wi.mit.edu/MPR`. Intensities were captured by the GeneChip^{TM} Software (Affymetrix, Santa Clara, CA) and were scaled so that the overall intensity for each chip was made constant across the set of arrays. For each gene, a trimmed mean of the intensity differences from the 20 probe pairs representing it on the array was calculated as its summary expression level. Tamayo et al. (1999) reported trimmed means of less than 20 as 20, and trimmed means greater than 20,000 as 20,000. The profile for each gene consisted of its summary expression measure recorded for each of the four timepoints.

Tamayo et al. (1999) filtered their data for self-organizing map clustering by excluding genes that did not exhibit substantial variation in expression measurements across the four timepoints. They required included genes to have a maximum/minimum expression level of at least 3 and a maximum-minimum expression level of at least 100. This left 585 genes for their self organizing map analysis.

B.6 Hedenfalk Breast Cancer Data

The data of Hedenfalk et al. (2001) consist of expression profiles of 22 breast tumors taken from 21 patients. Because the analysis of the publication is based on analysis of 22 tumors, we use all 22 expression profiles in the analyses in Chapter 9. Seven of the tumors were from patients with germline BRCA1 mutations, eight were from patients with germline BRCA2 tumors, and seven were from patients with neither BRCA1 nor BRCA2 germline mutations. RNA from the specimens was analyzed on an array consisting of 6512 cDNA spots representing 2905 known and 2456 unknown genes. The reference RNA was derived from the MCF-10A human mammary epithelial cell line. Normalized ratios were available for 3226 genes meeting quality standards of an average intensity of more than 2500, an average spot area of more than 40 pixels, and no more than one sample in which the size of the spot area was 0 pixels. Only normalized ratios were provided. Ratios were calculated as intensity for the tumor sample divided by intensity for internal reference and were then normalized using image processing software. The data were downloaded from http://research.nhgri.nih.gov/microarray/NEJM_Supplement/. We have taken logarithms to the base 2 in the dataset we provide.

Details about all datasets provided on the book Web site are given in Appendix C.

C
BRB-ArrayTools

C.1 Software Description

The datasets used in this book are available at http://linus.nci.nih.gov/BRB-ArrayTools.html. The reader is encouraged to analyze these data sets using whatever software with which he or she is most comfortable. For readers who do not have software, we provide information here about the BRB-ArrayTools package that implements many of the methods described in this book. More detailed information about BRB-ArrayTools is available in the Users Guide (Simon and Lam 2003). For noncommercial applications, BRB-ArrayTools can be obtained without charge at the Web site. The package can be licensed from NIH for commercial use by contacting the NIH Technology Transfer Office at the telephone number indicated on the Web site and a 60 day trial version is available.

BRB-ArrayTools is an integrated package for the analysis of DNA microarray data developed by Dr. Richard Simon and Ms. Amy Peng Lam. It is intended to be usable by biologists, and it contains sophisticated and powerful analytic and visualization tools that the statisticians in the Biometric Research Branch of the National Cancer Institute have found useful in their collaborations. Tools were selected based on substantial experience with the analysis of DNA microarray data, knowledge of statistical theory, and critical review of the burgeoning literature of methods for analysis. The package is an attempt to encapsulate good statistical practice and to facilitate the training of biologists in the analysis of their microarray data. Although no software package is a substitute for collaboration with a trained and experienced statistician, such individuals are in short supply.

BRB-ArrayTools is implemented as an add-in for Microsoft Excel 2000 and later versions for computers running the Microsoft Windows family of operating systems. Although most of the analytic and visualization tools are performed by backend programs external to Excel, the interface to backend programs is invisible to the user who only needs to interact with the special BRB-ArrayTools menu in Excel and with the dialog boxes programmed into Excel using Visual Basic for Applications. The system is very portable and easily extensible, important features in the diverse and dynamic world of DNA microarrays. The program can accommodate about 240 arrays and 50,000 genes per project. BRB-ArrayTools contains a plug-in feature that enables users and other methodologists to insert their own analysis tools in the program. The plug-in must be written in the powerful and popular R statistical language (available at the BRB-ArrayTools Web site). The plug-in facility provides a wizard enabling the R function developer to provide VBA dialog boxes for user interaction because the R language itself does not have an effective dialog capability. The wizard creates the dialog for the developer so the user does not need to know Visual Basic for Applications.

BRB-ArrayTools is applicable to data from dual-label glass arrays, Affymetrix GeneChips^{TM}, and filter arrays. The package operates on "spot" or "probe set" level data produced by image analysis programs and by the Affymetrix Microarray Analysis Suite software. Most users import into BRB-ArrayTools either the background-adjusted Cy3 and Cy5 intensities for each spot on a dual-label glass array, or the signal for each probe set on an Affymetrix GeneChip^{TM}. Importing spot flag indicators, spot size values, and background levels are optional. These data are usually given in a separate file for each array. There is a row for each spot or probe set and the columns represent the variables measured for that spot on that array. In this intensity file there must be some spot or probe set identifier, such as a probe set ID or a spot index. The identifier is used for two purposes: to align the rows of intensity files for the different arrays and to link the intensity data to additional spot identifier data that may be contained in a separate flat file containing optional columns such as Gene Title, clone ID, Genbank accession number, Unigene ID, and Gene Symbol. Not all of these identifiers need to be given, but providing at least one such identifier will enable the package to provide hyperlinked gene annotation information on spots that are identified as being of interest from the various analysis and visualization tools. For Affymetrix GeneChip^{TM} data, the probe set ID is usually the identifier in the expression data files and no other identifier or identifier file is needed. For dual-color glass arrays, the additional identifiers may occupy columns directly on each intensity file instead of being in a separate gene identifier file.

In addition to the files of intensity or signal data and the file of spot or probe set identifiers, the user must provide an experiment descriptor worksheet. The rows of this file correspond to the arrays to be analyzed. The first column of the experiment descriptor worksheet must provide the file name of the intensity data for the array corresponding to that row. The other columns provide user-determined descriptors of the arrays. The descriptors generally refer to features of the experimental specimens hybridized to the arrays. For example, in an analysis of breast tumor specimens, one column might contain indicators of which arrays correspond to estrogen-receptor positive tumors and which correspond to estrogen-receptor negative tumors. For dual-label arrays, it is usually assumed that one channel is a common internal reference RNA and the columns of the experiment descriptor worksheet refer to the experimental specimen in the other channel. Any coding of the descriptors can be used, but the spelling must be consistent. For example, one could code the column ER+ for the positive tumors and ER- for the negative tumors; one need not invent numerical codes. Tumors of unknown estrogen-receptor status would be blank in the ER column and would be omitted in any analysis comparing the ER+ to the ER- tumors. The experiment descriptor worksheet is used by BRB-ArrayTools to drive class comparison and class prediction analyses, to tell the program which arrays to use in analysis and which to omit, and to provide a mechanism for specifying how dendrograms and multidimensional scaling plots should be labeled and colored.

In some cases the user may wish to import expression data that have already been horizontally aligned and placed in a single file with each row corresponding to a spot or probe set and blocks of columns providing expression data for each array. BRB-ArrayTools provides this option. It is also possible to import dual-label glass slide data for which only the log ratios are available, and not the channel-specific intensities.

During the data import step, BRB-ArrayTools also performs filtering and normalization. Many of the options described in Chapters 5 and 6 are available. After the data have been imported, filtered, and normalized, the imported data are saved in a project workbook in Excel. The user may utilize the provided tools for analysis, then close the project workbook and leave Excel. At any later time the user can reopen Excel, open the project workbook, and resume the analysis by selecting additional tools.

More information about data importing and all aspects of BRB-ArrayTools is available from the Users Guide (Simon and Lam 2003) which can be found on the Web site.

C.2 Analysis of Bittner Melanoma Data

The melanoma data of Bittner et al. (2000) analyzed in Chapter 9 is described in Appendix B. The data provided by Bittner et al. (2000) are the ratios for the 3613 genes that were considered "well measured" because their intensities were sufficiently high. We have converted these ratios to $\log_2$ ratios. The $\log_2$ ratios for the 31 cDNA arrays resulting from analysis of 31 melanoma specimens are available in the file Bittner_expression.dat which contains 3614 rows and 34 columns. The first row is a header that contains column labels. Each of the other rows corresponds to one of the well-measured genes. The first column contains a clone identifier, the second column contains the Unigene cluster identifier, and the third column contains a gene title. A very rudimentary experiment descriptor file, named Bittner_exp_description.dat, is also provided. It contains a header row followed by 31 rows corresponding to the 31 arrays. The rows of the experiment descriptor file correspond to the arrays in the horizontally aligned expression data file and they are in the same order. The first column of the experiment descriptor file contains array names. The second column contains a specimen number (1 to 31) used in Chapter 9 for the analysis of these data. The last column indicates which specimens were found to be part of the cluster identified by Bittner et al. (2000) and by the analysis presented in Chapter 9. This column would not, of course, have been part of the experiment descriptor file at the time of initial analysis, but is provided here for convenience in labeling dendrograms.

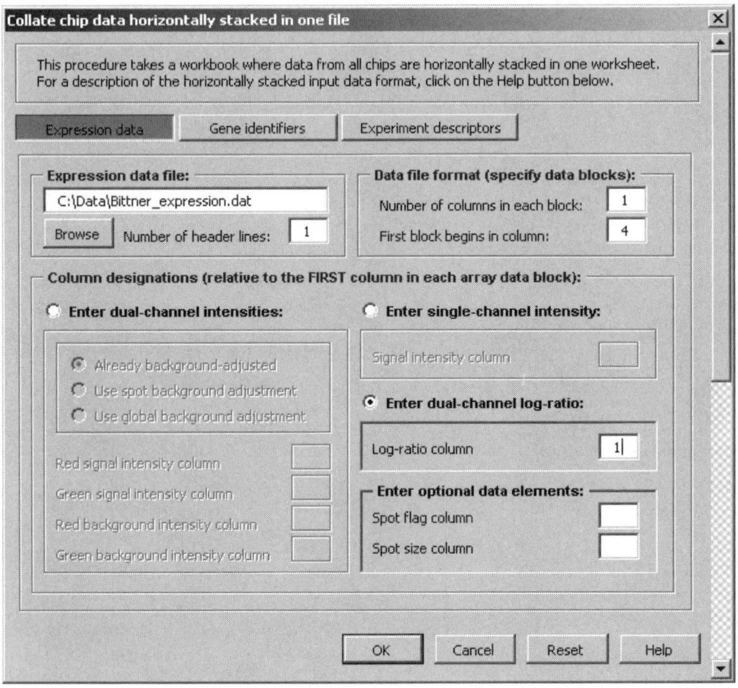

Fig. C.1. BRB-ArrayTools dialog box expression data tab for collation of Bittner melanoma data.

Figure C.1 shows the first BRB-ArrayTools dialog for collating horizontally aligned data. The dialog boxes sometimes change with new releases of BRB-ArrayTools, so the dialog boxes you see with your BRB-ArrayTools software may not agree exactly with those illustrated here. This box requests information about the expression data file. There is a browse button to enable the user to find the file containing the horizontally aligned expression levels. For horizontally aligned data, it is assumed that the data for the different arrays are in contiguous blocks of columns but there may be multiple columns of information for each array. For the melanoma data there is actually only a single column of information for each array, the $\log_2$ ratio. In other cases, however, the information may include Cy5 intensity, Cy3 intensity, spot size, spot flag, and so on. The two fields under "Data file format" are filled in to indicate that for these data there is only one column per block and that the block for the first array starts in column 4 of the file. The first three columns of the file contain clone identification information. The button for "Enter dual channel log ratios" is selected to indicate that only the log ratios, not the channel-specific intensities are available. When this is the case, the dialog under "Enter dual channel intensities" is greyed out. The log ratio column is indicated as column 1 because it is the first (and only) column in each block of information for each array. The optional spot size and spot filter fields are blank because that information is not available. If it were available, the column numbers we would indicate would be column numbers relative to the first column of a block.

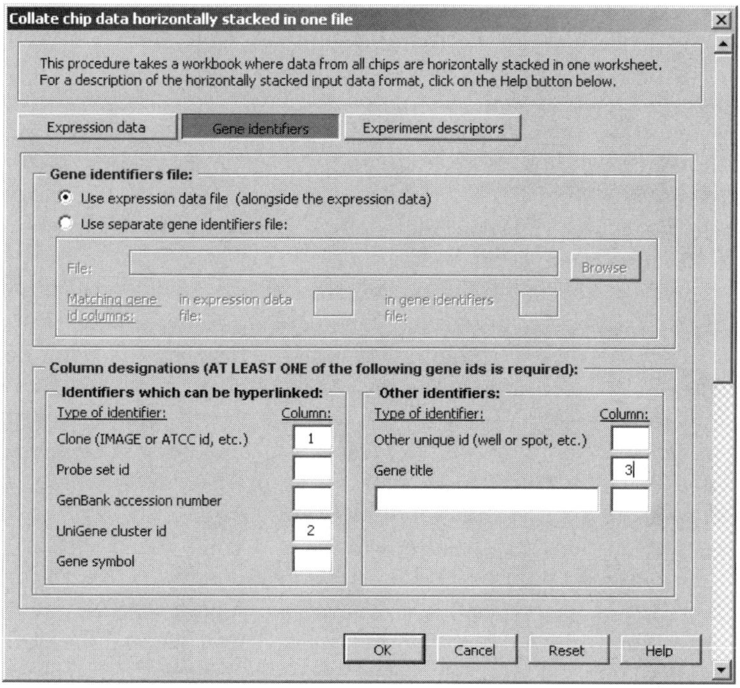

Fig. C.2. BRB-ArrayTools dialog box gene identifiers tab for collation of Bittner melanoma data.

After completing the "Expression data" tab, you should select the "Gene identifiers" tab shown in Figure C.2. The gene identifier information can either be in the initial columns of the file containing the expression data, or in a separate file. For the melanoma data, they are in the first three columns of the file containing the expression data. In this case there are only three identifiers. The first column is the IMAGE Consortium clone identifier. The second column is the Unigene cluster identifier, and the third column is a gene title as indicated in the figure.

The third tab requests information about the experiment descriptor file. You can browse to indicate the complete path of the file. For dual-label arrays, most of the analysis tools of BRB-ArrayTools assume that a reference design has been used. That is, it is assumed that all of the experimental samples have been cohybridized with a common reference RNA specimen, and that the same label has been used for the reference on each array. If the labeling of the reference and the experimental specimen are reversed for some arrays, then the button "Flip ratios on reverse fluor experiments" should be selected and you should then indicate what column of the experiment descriptor file indicates which arrays were labeled "forward" and which "reverse".

After completing the three dialog tabs to provide information about the expression data, the gene descriptors, and the experiment descriptor file, you are presented with a dialog for filtering and normalization. There are three tabs of filter information. The first is for filtering spots that have low intensities, small sizes (in pixels), or spots that have been flagged as unreliable by the image analysis program or by visual inspection of the images. For the melanoma data, we do not have channel-specific intensities, spot sizes, or flag values, so we do not select any of these filters. The melanoma data made available by Bittner et al. (2000) include only spots that were considered "well measured" and so were prefiltered.

The second tab of the filter dialog enables you to exclude genes that either did not show much variability among the arrays or which were filtered from too many arrays because of low intensity or other problems. It is not necessary to filter the genes at all unless one wishes to cluster the genes. Hierarchical clustering of genes is memory intensive, as similarity of expression profiles for all pairs of genes needs to be computed. For gene clustering it is generally best to first omit the genes that do not show substantial variation among samples and those that are not well measured on many arrays.

One option provided for the filter criteria is to filter based on the variation in the log ratio or log signal value. The variance is computed for each gene over the complete set of arrays. One might wish to compare that variance to that of a housekeeping gene and to filter the gene if its variance is not statistically significantly greater. Because the variance for a housekeeping gene is often not known, the median of the variance values for all genes is used as the variance expected for a housekeeping gene. This is based on the assumption that most of the genes are not differentially expressed among the arrays. Another option is to select the genes with the greatest variances; the proportion of the genes selected can be indicated in the dialog. A third option is to filter genes for which the proportion of arrays in which the expression differs from the median expression (for that gene) by less than a specified-fold difference is below a threshold level. The dialog also permits you to indicate how many arrays the gene can be filtered from before the gene is excluded entirely. For this analysis we have not requested any gene filtering.

The normalization tab permits you to indicate whether you want the data to be normalized. In general, the answer will be yes. For the melanoma data, however, the data were previously normalized and not all of the genes are provided, hence we specify that the data should not be renormalized. When channel-specific intensities are provided for dual-label data, two normalization options are available: normalizing to make the median log ratio on each array zero, and intensity-dependent loess normalization as described in Chapter 5. When only log ratios are provided, intensity-dependent normalization is not possible. For Affymetrix GeneChip^{TM} data, the arrays are normalized by computing for each array the log ratios of signal values relative to signal values for the first array in the experiment descriptor file. A normalization constant is determined for each array to make the median of these log ratios zero, where the median is either computed over the specified housekeeping genes or over all the genes if housekeeping genes are not available.

The normalization dialog also provides the option of truncating extreme ratio values for dual-label arrays that are likely to be outliers.

After completing the normalization dialog, you should click the ok button and then click the ok button for the main collation dialog. The collation, filtering and normalization are then performed. BRB-ArrayTools will also try to download annotation information for the genes on your array if you have given it sufficient gene identification information and are connected to the Internet when you do the collation. This entire process may take several minutes, particularly the download of gene annotation information. When the collation is completed, your project workbook is created. You may close this workbook at any time and come back to it at a later time by opening the project workbook and selecting more analyses to run from BRB-ArrayTools.

The objective of the melanoma study by Bittner et al. (2000) was to discover whether there were subsets of patients with advanced disease that could be identified by their gene expression profiles. Although some class comparison analyses were carried out, the dominant focus was on class discovery. BRB-ArrayTools contains two types of tools for addressing this objective. One is the tool for hierarchical clustering of samples. When this is selected from the menu, the dialog box shown in Figure C.3 appears. There are many clustering algorithms and clustering is an exploratory and subjective method of analysis. BRB-ArrayTools offers only hierarchical clustering, but even within this there are several options that must be specified, as described in Chapter 9. Figure C.3 shows that for the analysis of the melanoma samples we have requested average linkage hierarchical clustering using the centered correlation similarity metric using as the expression values the log$_2$ ratios. We have not requested median centering of the genes. All of the genes not excluded by gene filtering during collation are used in computing the similarity metric, and all of the arrays are included in the analysis. You could perform the clustering using only a subset of genes contained in a gene list if you wanted. The dialog also asks you whether you wish the program to compute cluster reproducibility measures, as described in Chapter 9.

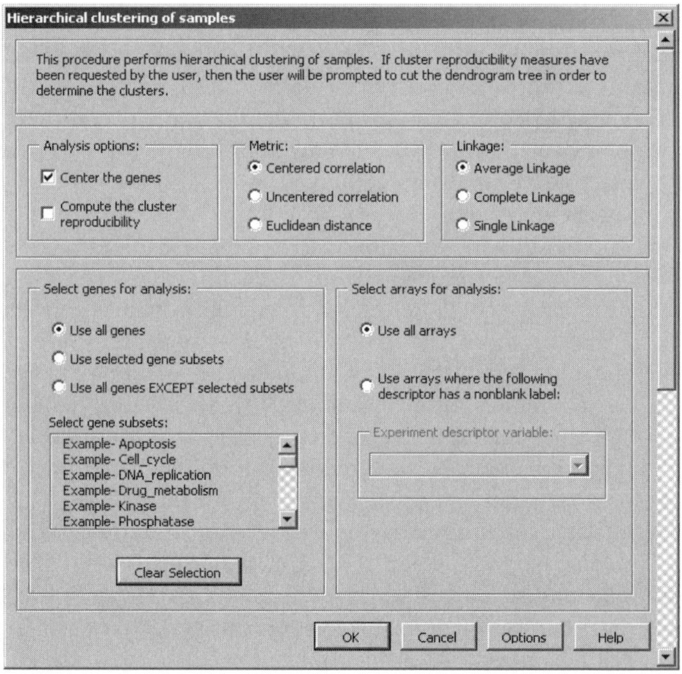

Fig. C.3. BRB-ArrayTools dialog box for cluster analysis of samples on Bittner melanoma data.

Before pressing the ok button, you should press the options button. On the options dialog you can specify how you would like the samples labeled in the dendrogram that the tool will produce. The dialog shows you the column headings from your experiment design worksheet, and you select one of the columns for labeling. For your reanalysis of these data, it is useful to use the third column of the experiment descriptor worksheet for labeling the dendrogram. This column indicates specimens belonging to the cluster of interest identified by Bittner et al. (2000). The options dialog also requests specification of how many times the data should be randomly perturbed for calculating the cluster reproducibility estimates; the default value is 100. It also requests the standard deviation that should be used for the random perturbations. If the assay standard deviation is not known from reproducibility studies, the tool will compute the standard deviation for all genes and use the median value as the assay standard deviation.

After pressing the ok button for the options dialog and the ok button for the hierarchical clustering of samples dialog, the analysis proceeds. The results produced include a dendrogram of the samples, labeled as requested on the options dialog, and the cluster reproducibility results. For computing cluster reproducibility, you must specify where to cut the dendrogram to give specific clusters. You are interactively prompted to do so if you have requested cluster reproducibility analyses. For the melanoma data, the dendrogram should look like the average linkage dendrogram in Figure 9.5 of Chapter 9. If you cut the dendrogram at a point corresponding to eight clusters (Table 9.2), the cluster reproducibility results you obtain should indicate that the cluster consisting of samples 6 to 24 is very reproducible within the context of this clustering algorithm.

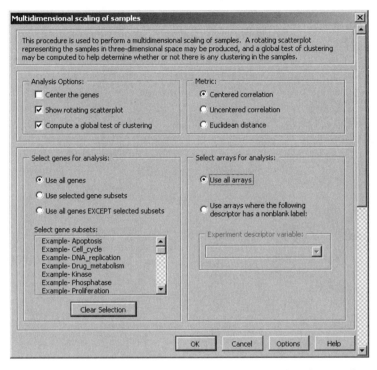

Fig. C.4. BRB-ArrayTools dialog box for multidimensional scaling analysis of Bittner melanoma data.

A second approach to class discovery in the melanoma data is use of the multidimensional scaling tool. The multidimensional scaling dialog is shown in Figure C.4. It is similar to the dialog for hierarchical clustering of samples. The two outputs of this tool are a rotating 3-D scatterplot in which each sample is represented by a point in the scatterplot. The user has control of the speed and direction of rotation and can use those controls to try to identify views that show clusters of samples. The dimensions of the display are the three linear combinations of the genes that are orthogonal to each other and that provide a 3-D representation that best preserves the distances between the samples in the original high-dimensional space of the gene expression vectors (Section 9.3.1). The rotating scatterplot can be stopped by the user. Points can be selected for identification by brushing the points with the mouse while holding down the left mouse button. The identities of the samples corresponding to the brushed points are identified below the scatterplot. The rotating 3-D scatterplot can also be imported into a Powerpoint presentation for display on a computer with the BRB-ArrayTools software.

The points on the multidimensional scaling plot represent specimens. They are color-coded based on a column of the experiment descriptor worksheet specified by the user on the options dialog page that is reached by pressing the options button on the multidimensional scaling dialog. The options page also requests the user to specify how many random permutations (default 1000) to perform in computing the statistical significance test of the null hypothesis that the samples are not clustered in 3-D space more than would be expected for a multivariate normal distribution (see Section 9.5.1). On the multidimensional scaling dialog, you specify the distance metric to use for measuring distance between expression profiles of each pair of samples. For the melanoma data, the 3-D projections of the expression profiles are significantly different from what one would expect for a multivariate normal distribution. As indicated in Chapter 9, the statistical significance level is approximately 0.01 when using centered correlations of noncentered genes as the distance metric.

C.3 Analysis of Perou Breast Cancer Chemotherapy Data

The Perou breast cancer dataset is described in Appendix B and represents published microarray expression profiles of 20 breast tumors before and after chemotherapy. These data were analyzed in Chapter 7.

File Perou_expression.dat provides the intensity data for all arrays horizontally aligned with each line of the file giving all the data for each of the 9217 clones represented on the array. The first five columns of the file contain a gene title, clone type indicator, Genbank accession number, IMAGE clone identifier, and spot index, respectively. The remaining columns contain the actual array data, arranged in 40 blocks of 3 columns per block. Each block corresponds to an array. The columns within a block are the Cy3 signal (foreground minus background), Cy5 signal, and a flag column. A flag value other than zero indicates that the intensity data were considered not reliable.

File Perou_exp_description.dat is the experiment descriptor file prepared for this dataset. It contains 41 rows, a header row and a row for each of the 40 arrays. The first column contains identifiers for the arrays. The second column contains identifiers for the patients whose breast tumor specimens were hybridized to the arrays. A reference design was used and the tumors were always labeled with Cy5. The internal reference was a mixture of cell lines. Tumors were biopsied both before and after the patient received chemotherapy. The third column contains indicators of whether the array corresponds to a tumor sampled before ("BE") or after ("AF") chemotherapy.

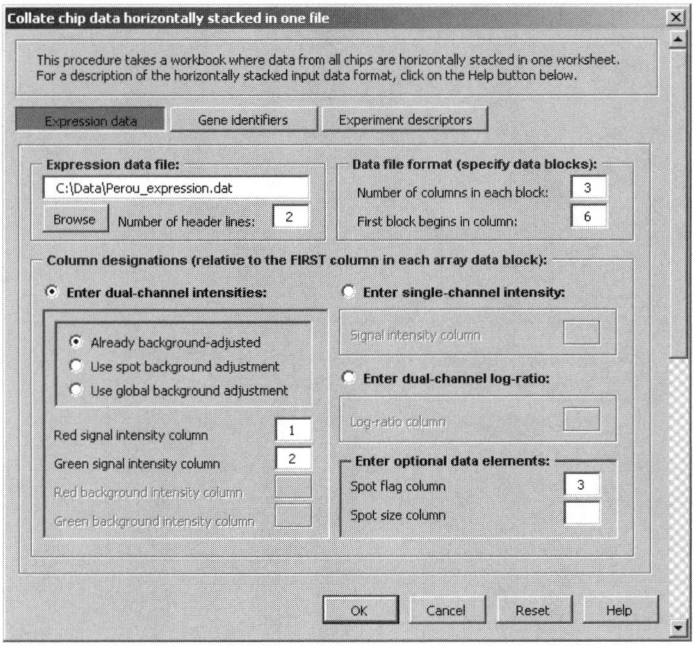

Fig. C.5. BRB-ArrayTools dialog box expression data tab for collation of Perou breast cancer chemotherapy data.

The data can be imported into BRB-ArrayTools using the "collate horizontally aligned data" tool. The intensity and gene dialog boxes are filled in as shown in Figures C.5 and C.6. The file names have to be adjusted based on the names and locations you have given to these files after you downloaded them. Note that the expression data file has two header rows, not the one which is the default in the dialog box. The data are filtered in the following way. If the background-adjusted intensities in both channels are less than 100, then the information is filtered out. If one channel is less than 100 and the other is above 100, then the spot is not filtered, but the ratio is calculated after bringing the smaller value up to 100. Spots with a flag field other than zero are also filtered. The spot size filter is not used inasmuch as spot size is not included in the imported data fields. The genes were filtered only for excluding genes whose expression levels are missing or filtered in more than 10 arrays. The analysis in Chapter 7 excluded spots that were missing in either pre- or posttreatment specimens from more than 10 patients. BRB-ArrayTools does not provide this option. Consequently the number of spots passing the filter is 8065 for the data collated by BRB-ArrayTools compared to 8029 in Chapter 7. We normalized the data by centering the median log ratios on each array. Ratios greater than 64 or less than 1/64 were replaced by the default thresholds of 64 and 1/64, respectively.

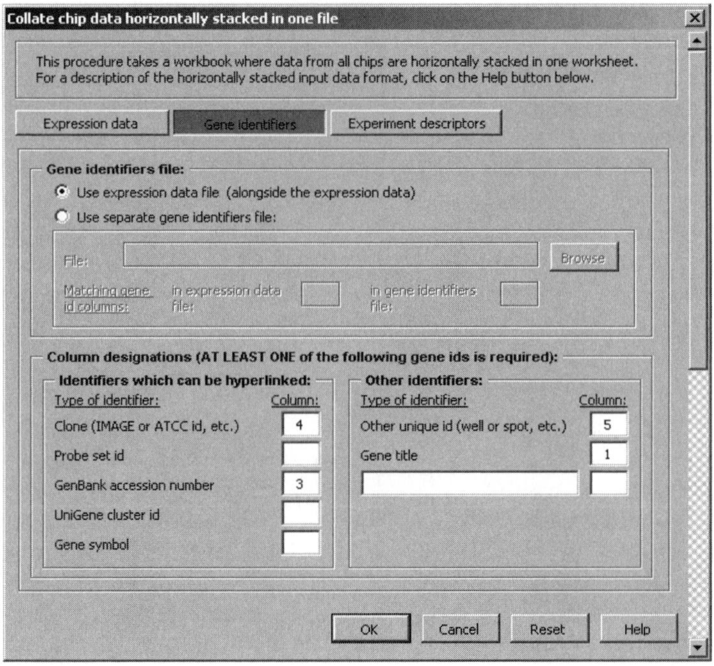

Fig. C.6. BRB-ArrayTools dialog box gene identifiers tab for collation of Perou breast cancer chemotherapy data.

Our objective in analyzing the Perou et al. (2000) data was to identify genes that were differentially expressed in the prechemotherapy specimens compared to the postchemotherapy specimens. This can be addressed using the class comparison tool in the classification menu. The emphasis here is on identifying differentially expressed genes, not on prediction, so the class comparison tool is more appropriate than the class prediction tool. The class comparison dialog is shown in Figure C.7. The arrays are paired for this analysis, because a before chemotherapy and after chemotherapy expression profile is available for each patient. This is indicated in the dialog and you browse for the "Patient ID" label to indicate the column of the experiment descriptor file that indicates which arrays correspond to the same patient. You also indicate that the classes to be compared are defined by the column of the experiment descriptor worksheet labeled "BeforeAfter".

BRB-ArrayTools contains several methods for controlling the number of false positive claims that genes are differentially expressed. The user has the option of selecting the methods to be used. Generally it is advisable to select all the methods. As shown in Figure C.7, we have requested that gene lists be produced based on all of the criteria: univariate significance level less than 0.001, number of false discoveries less than 5, and proportion of false discoveries less than 10%. In the output, a single gene list will be produced.

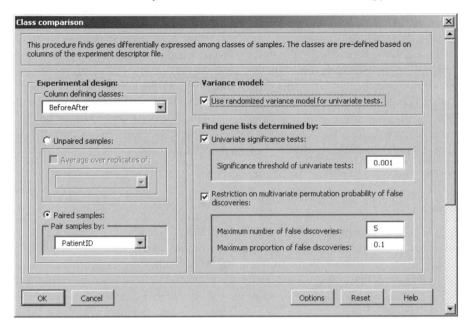

Fig. C.7. BRB-ArrayTools dialog box for class comparison analysis of Perou breast cancer chemotherapy data.

The gene list will be ordered by the univariate parametric significance levels. The gene list should be truncated at different points, however, depending on which of the criteria is of interest. This truncation information is provided at the top of the output file. In the example, there are 65 genes that satisfy the univariate significance less than 0.001 criterion (the first 65 rows of the gene list). The output indicates how many genes in the gene list should be included in order to satisfy the criterion of limiting the number or proportion of false discoveries using the multivariate permutation tests described in Chapter 7. In order to have the median number of false discoveries equal to 5, the first 79 genes on the output should be considered the appropriate gene list. In order to have 95% confidence that the number of false discoveries does not exceed 5, the gene list should consist of the first 37 genes. The program also computes the gene list for controlling the proportion of false discoveries. In order to have the median proportion of false discoveries equal 10%, the gene list should consist of the first 118 genes on the output. In order to have 95% confidence that the proportion of false discoveries does not exceed 10% the gene list should consist of the first 27 genes.

Because the multivariate permutation tests are nonparametric and more powerful than the univariate permutation tests, it is generally not necessary to request the latter in the options dialog.

The dialog shown in Figure C.7 provides the option of using a "Randomized Variance t-test" instead of the usual t-test. The Randomized Variance method is described by Wright and Simon (2003) and is similar to the method described by Baldi and Long (2001). It makes the assumption that the within-class variances for all genes represent random draws from a common probability distribution, but not that the variances are the same for different genes (Section 7.4). Because it provides for some sharing of information among genes, it is more efficient for studies with few samples per class. If the Randomized Variance option is selected, it is used for ordering the gene list, for the permutation tests, and for determining how many genes satisfy the false discovery number and false discovery rate criteria.

C.4 Analysis of Hedenfalk Breast Cancer Data

The breast cancer data of Hedenfalk et al. (2001) analyzed in Chapter 8 are described in Appendix B. The only data provided by Hedenfalk et al. (2001) are the ratios of intensities for tumor samples divided by internal reference for the 3226 genes that were considered well measured. We have converted these ratios to $\log_2$ ratios. The $\log_2$ ratios for the 22 cDNA arrays are available in the file BRCA_expression.dat. The first three rows are headers. The first three columns contain clone information and the remaining 22 columns are the $\log_2$ ratios for the 22 tumor specimens. The first three columns contain inventory well/plate identifier, IMAGE clone identifier, and gene title, respectively.

The file BRCA_exper.dat is an experiment descriptor file for use with these data. The rows are ordered to correspond to the columns of the expression data. The first column of the experiment descriptor file gives a patient index and the second column gives a specimen identifier. The third column gives the mutation status of the specimen. The final three columns give binary groupings of the mutation status; BRCA1 mutated or not, BRCA2 mutated or not, and sporadic or not. For developing a class predictor of whether the specimen is derived from a patient with a germline BRCA2 mutation, we use the column labeled "BRCA2 ?".

The data are collated (e.g., imported) to BRB-ArrayTools as described for the melanoma data. Only log ratios are available, therefore several of the filtering and normalization options are not available. The log ratios provided were previously normalized. Because not all of the genes are provided, the data should not be renormalized.

The main objectives of the analysis of the BRCA data were class comparison and class prediction. We have already illustrated the class comparison tool with the Perou data, therefore here we describe the class prediction tool. In Chapter 8 this dataset was used to illustrate developing a predictor of whether a sample was derived from a patient with a germline BRCA2 mutation. The class prediction dialog is illustrated in Figure C.8. We have selected the column describing the class variable to be the one in the experiment descriptor file that distinguishes BRCA2 mutated from BRCA2 nonmutated specimens.

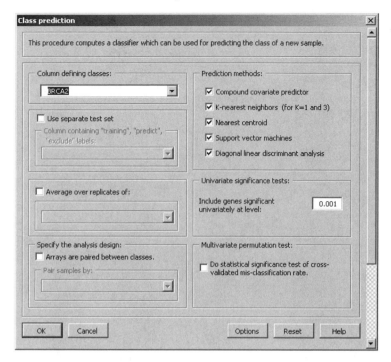

Fig. C.8. BRB-ArrayTools dialog box for class prediction analysis of Hedenfalk germline BRCA mutation data.

Our specimens are not paired. We have indicated that we want feature selection to be based on genes that are differentially expressed between the classes with a parametric t-test $p < 0.001$. The dialog permits us to specify the predictive models we would like to study. The default is to develop all of the types permitted. The options include diagonal linear discriminant analysis, compound covariate predictor, k-nearest neighbor classifier for k=1 and k=3; nearest centroid classifier, and support vector machine with linear kernel.

The class prediction dialog permits us to designate samples that we wish to exclude from the analysis. The excluded samples may represent samples whose classification is unknown. When the analysis is complete and all leave-one-out cross-validations have been performed, the tool will provide a class prediction for each excluded sample using for prediction each type of model selected. The prediction is based on the models fitted to all of the nonexcluded samples. Whereas leave-one-out cross-validation is used to obtain an unbiased estimate of the misclassification rate, prediction for future samples is best based on a model fitted using the entire set of nonexcluded samples. The excluded samples may represent a separate set of test samples whose true classification is unknown. The user may also indicate that some of the samples are to be excluded and no prediction for them is desired. These features are described in more detail in the BRB-ArrayTools User's Guide.

Leave-one-out cross-validation is performed. For each leave-one-out training set, the genes that are differentially expressed between the two classes by a t-test at the specified level (e.g., $p < 0.001$) in the training set are determined. All of the specified models are built in that training set for that gene set, and the class of the left-out sample is predicted. This is repeated, leaving out one sample at a time, and the cross-validated misclassification rate for each method is determined. If requested, the entire cross-validation process can be repeated many times with randomly permuted class labels in order to determine the proportion of the time with random permutations one obtains a cross-validated misclassification rate as small as obtained with the real data. This is the statistical significance level associated with the cross-validated misclassification rate. This significance level is computed for each classification method studied. Not requesting the statistical significance test does not affect the computation of the cross-validated misclassification rates. Computing the statistical significance level is much more time consuming.

The cross-validated misclassification rates and associated statistical significance levels are reported in an output html file. The file indicates the prediction of each sample for each method. The output file also gives the set of predictor genes that meet the feature selection criteria when applied to the full dataset. The gene set differs for each leave-one-out training set and one column of the output file indicates the proportion of the leave-one-out training sets in which each gene is contained.

References

Adams R and Bischof L. (1994) Seeded region growing. *IEEE Trans. Pattern Anal. Mach.* Intell. 16:641-647.

Affymetrix (2001a) *Statistical Algorithms Reference Guide.* Santa Clara, CA; Affymetrix 2001.

Affymetrix, (2000) *GeneChip*^{TM} *Expression Analysis.* Technical manual.

Affymetrix. (2001b) *Affymetrix Microarray Suite User Guide, Version 5.* Santa Clara, CA; Affymetrix.

Affymetrix. (2002) GeneChip^{TM} Expression Analysis Data Analysis Fundamentals. Available at http://www.affymetrix.com/support/technical/manuals.affx.

Alizadeh AA, Eisen MB, Davis RE, Ma C, Lossos IS, Rosenwald A, Boldrick JC, Sabet H, Tran T, Yu X, Powell JI, Yang L, Marti GE, Moore T, Hudson Jr. J, Lu L, Lewis DB, Tibshirani R, Sherlock G, Cahn WC, Greiner TC, Weisenburger DD, Armitage JO, Warnke R, Levy R, Wilson W, Grever MR, Byrd JC, Botstein D, Brown PO, and Staudt LM. (2000) Different types of diffuse large B-cell lymphoma identified by gene expression profiling. *Nature* 403:503-511.

Ambroise C and McLachlan GJ. (2002) Selection bias in gene extraction on the basis of microarray gene expression data. *Proc. Nati. Acad. Sci. USA.*

Aronow BJ, Richardson BD, and Handwerger, S. (2001) Microarray analysis of trophoblast differentiation: gene expression reprogramming in key gene function categories. *Physiol. Genomics*, 6, 2: 105-116.

Assersohn L, Gangi L, Zhao Y, Dowsett M, Simon R, Powles TJ, and Liu ET. (2002) The feasibility of using fine needle aspiration from primary breast cancers for cDNA microarray analyses. *Clin. Cancer Res.* 8: 794-801.

Axon Instruments, Inc. (2001) *GenePix Pro 4.0 User's Guide.*

Baldi P and Long AD. (2001) A Bayesian framework for the analysis of microarray expression data: Regularized *t*-test and statistical inferences of gene changes. Bioinf. 17: 509-519.

Banfield JD and Raftery AE. (1992) Model-based Gaussian and non-Gaussian clustering. *Biometrics*, 49: 803-822.

Ben-Dor A, Friedman N, and Yakhini Z. (2001) Class discovery in gene expression data. In *Proceedings of the Fifth Annual International Conference on Computational Molecular Biology, New York*: Association of Computing Machinery.

Benjamini Y and Hochberg Y. (1995). Controlling the false discovery rate: A practical and powerful approach to multiple testing. *J. Roy. Stati. Soc., Ser. B*, 57: 289-300.

Beucher S and Meyer F. (1993) The morphological approach to segmentation: The water shed transformation. *In Mathematical Morphology in Image Processing*, vol. 34 of Optical Engineering, New York: Marcel Dekker, pp. 443-481.

Bittner M, Meltzer P, Chen Y, Jiang Y, Seftor E, Hendrix M, Radmacher M, Simon R, Yakhini Z, Ben-Dor A, Dougherty E, Wang E, Marincola F, Gooden C, Lueders J, Glatfelter A, Pollock P, Gillanders E, Leja D, Dietrich K, Beaudry C, Berens M, Alberts D, Sondak V, Hayward N, and Trent J. (2000) Molecular classification of cutaneous malignant melanoma by gene expression profiling. *Nature*, 406, 536-540.

Black MA and Doerge RW. (2002) Calculation of the minimum number of replicate spots required for detection of significant gene expression fold change in microarray experiments. *Bioinf.* 18:1609-1616.

Bolstad B. (2001) Probe Level Quantile Normalization of High Density Oligonucleotide Array. Unpublished manuscript. Available at `http://stat-www.berkeley.edu/~bolstad/stuff/qnorm.pdf`.

Bolstad BM, Irizarry RA, Astrand M, and Speed TP. (2003) A comparison of normalization methods for high density array data based on variance and bias. *Bioinf.* 19:185-193.

Breiman L. (1996) Bagging predictors. *Mach. Learn.* 24:123-140.

Breiman L. (1998) Arcing classifiers. *Ann. Stat.* 26:801-824.

Breiman L, Friedman J, Stone C, and Olshen R. (1984) *Classification and Regression Trees*, Belmont, CA: Wadsworth.

Brody JP, William BA, Wold BJ, and Quake SR. (2002) Significance and statistical errors in the analysis of DNA microarray data, *Proc. Nat. Acad. Sci. USA* 99:12975-12978.

Broet P, Richardson S, and Radvanyi F. (2002) Bayesian hierarchical model for identifying changes in gene expression from microarray experiments. *J. Comput. Biol.* 9:671-683.

Brown CS, Goodwin PC, and Sorger PK. (2001) Image metrics in the statistical analysis of DNA microarray data. *Proc. Nat. Acad. Sci. USA* 98:8944-8949.

Brown MPS, Grundy WN, Lin D, Cristianini N, Sugnet CW, Furey TS, Ares M Jr. and Haussler D. (2000) Knowledge-based analysis of microarray gene expression data by using support vector machines. *Proc. Nat. Acad. Sci. USA* 97:262-267.

Callow MJ, Dudoit S, Gong EL, Speed TP, and Rubin EM. (2000) Microarray expression profiling identifies genes with altered expression in HDL-deficient mice. *Genome Res.* 10: 2022-2029.

Chee M, Yang Y, Hubbell E, Berno A, Huang XC, Stern D, Winkler J, Lockhart DJ, Morris MS, and Fodor SPA.(1996) Accessing genetic information with high-density DNA arrays. *Science* 274: 610-614.

Chen, Y, Dougherty ER, and Bittner ML. (1997) Ratio-based decisions and the quantitative analysis of cDNA microarray images. *J. Biomed. Optics* 2:364-374.

Chen Y, Kamat V, Dougherty ER, Bittner ML, Meltzer PS, and Trent JM. (2002) Ratio statistics of gene expression levels and applications to microarray data analysis. *Bioinf.* 18:1207-1215.

Cheng Y and Church GM. (2000) Biclustering of expression data. *ISMB 2000*, 93-103.

Chung JH and Fraser DAS. (1958) Randomization tests for a multivariate two-sample problem. *J. Am. Stat. Assoc.* 53: 729-735.

Cox DR. (1970) *Analysis of Binary Data.* London: Methuen .

DeRisi J, Penland L, Brown PO, Bittner ML, Melzer PS, Ray M, Chen Y, Su YA, and Trent JM. (1996) Use of a cDNA microarray to analyze gene expression patterns in human cancer. *Nature Genetics* 14: 457-460.

DeRisi JL, Iyer VR, and Brown PO. (1997) The metabolic and genetic control of gene expression on a genomic scale. *Science* 278:680-686.

Desu MM and Raghavarao D. (1990) *Sample Size Methodology.* Boston: Academic Press.

Dobbin K and Simon R. (2002). Comparison of microarray designs for class comparison and class discovery. *Bioinf.* 18:1438-1445.

Dobbin K, Shih J, and Simon R. (2003a) Statistical design of reverse dye microarrays. *Bioinf.* 19: 803-810.

Dobbin K. Shih J, and Simon R. (2003b). Questions and answers on design of dual-label microarrays for identifying differentially expressed genes. *J. Nat. Cancer Inst.* 95:1362-69.

Draper NR and Smith H. (1998) *Applied Regression Analysis* 3rd ed. New York: Wiley.

Dudoit S. and Fridlyand J. (2002) A prediction-based resampling method for estimating the number of clusters in a dataset. *Genome Biol.* 3(7): 1-36.

Dudoit S, Fridlyad F, and Speed TP. (2002) Comparison of discrimination methods for classification of tumors using DNA microarrays. *J. Am. Stat. Assoc.* 97:77-87.

Efron B. (1983) Estimating the error rate of a prediction rule: Improvement on cross-validation. *J. Am. Stat. Assoc.* 78:316-331.

Efron B and Tibshirani R. (1997) Improvements on cross-validation: The .632+ bootstrap method. *J. Am. Stat. Assoc.* 92:548-560.

Efron B and Tibshirani RJ. (1998). *An Introduction To The Bootstrap* New York: Chapman & Hall/CRC, pp. 202-210.

Efron B, Tibshirani R, Storey JD, and Tusher V. (2001) Empirical Bayes analysis of a microarray experiment. *J. Am. Stat. Assoc.* 96:1151-1160.

Eisen MB and Brown PO. (1998) DNA arrays for analysis of gene expression. *Meth. Enzymol.* 303:179-205.

Eisen MB, Spellman PT, Brown PO, and Botstein D. (1998) Cluster analysis and display of genome-wide expression patterns. *Proc. Nat. Acad. Sci. USA* 95:14863-14868.

Fisher RA. (1936) The use of multiple measurements in taxonomic problems. *Ann. Eugenics* 7:179-188.

Fodor SPA, Read JL, Pirrung MC, Stryer L, Lu AT, and Solas D. (1991) Light-directed, spatially addressable parallel chemical synthesis. *Science* 251:767-773.

Fowlkes EB and Mallows CL. (1983) A method for comparing two hierarchical clusterings. *J. Am. Stat. Assoc.* 78, 553-569.

Furey TS, Cristianini N, Duffy N, Bednarski DW, Schummer M, and Haussler D. (2000) Support vector machine classification and validation of cancer tissue samples using microarray expression data. *Bioinf.*16: 906-914.

Gibbons FD and Roth FP. (2002) Judging the quality of gene expression-based clustering methods using gene annotation. *Genome Res.* 12, 1574-1581.

Gnanadesikan R, Kettenring JR, and Landwehr JM. (1977) Interpreting and assessing the results of cluster analysis. *Bull. Int. Stat. Inst.* 47: 451-463.

Golub T, Slonim D, Tamayo P, Huard C, Gaasenbeek M, Mesirov J, Coller H, Loh M, Dowing J, Caligiuri M, Bloomfield C, and Lander E. (1999) Molecular classification of cancer: Class discovery and class prediction by gene expression monitoring. *Science* 286:531-537.

Gordon AD. (1999) *Classification. (2nd ed.).* London: Chapman Hall/CRC.

Goryachev AB, Macgregor PF, Edwards AM. (2001) Unfolding of microarray data. *J. Comput. Biol.* 8: 443-461.

Harper CW. (1978) Groupings by locality in community ecology and paleoecology: Test of significance. *Lethaia,* 11: 251-257.

Harrell FE Jr, Califf RM, Pryor DB, Lee KL, and Rosati RA. (1982) Evaluating the yield of medical tests. *JAMA* 247:2543-2546.

Harrell FE Jr. (2001) *Regression Modeling Strategies.* New York: Springer.

Hastie T, Tibshirani R, and Friedman J. (2001) *The Elements of Statistical Learning: Data Mining, Inference and Prediction.* New York: Springer.

Hastie T, Tibshirani R, Eisen MB, Alizadeh A, Levy R, Staudt L Chan WC, Botstein D, and Brown PO. (2000) 'Gene shaving' as a method for identifying distinct sets of genes with similar expression patterns. *Genome Biol.* 1 (2), research0003.1-research0003.21.

Hedenfalk I, Duggan D, Chen Y, Radmacher M, Bittner M, Simon R, Meltzer P, Gusterson B, Esteller M, Kallioniemi O, Borg A, and Trent J. (2001) Gene expression profiles of hereditary breast cancer. *N. Eng. J. Med.* 344:549-548.

Hills M. (1966) Allocation rules and their error rates. J. Roy. Stat. Soc. *Ser. B.* 28:1-31.

Hoaglin DC, Mosteller F, and Tukey JW. (1983) *Understanding Robust and Exploratory Data Analysis.* New York; Wiley.

Hochberg Y. (1988) A sharper Bonferroni procedure for multiple tests of significance. *Biometrika* 75: 800-802.

Hollander M and Wolfe DA. (1999) *Nonparametric Statistical Methods*, 2nd Ed. New York: Wiley.

Holm S. (1979) A simple sequentially rejective multiple test procedure. *Scand. J. Stat.* 6:65-70.

Hotelling H. (1933) Analysis of a complex of statistical variables into principal components. *J. Ed. Psych.* 24: 417-441.

Hubbell E. (2001) Estimating signal with next generation Affymetrix software. In *Proceedings of the Gene Logic Workshop on Low Level Analysis of Affymetrix GeneChip*^{TM} *Data.* http://stat-www.berkeley.edu/users/terry/zarray/Affy/GL_Workshop/genelogic2001.html.

Hwang D, Schmitt WA, Stephanopoulos G, and Stephanopoulos G. (2002) Determination of minimum sample size and discriminatory expression patterns in microarray data. *Bioinf.* 18:1184-1193.

Irizarry RA, Hobbs B, Collin F, Beazer-Barclay YD, Antonellis KJ, Scherf U and Speed TP. (2003) Exploration, normalization, and summaries of high density oligonucleotide array probe level data. *Biostatistics* 4:249-264.

Jain AK and Dubes RC. (1988) *Algorithms for Clustering Data.* Englewood Cliffs, NJ: Prentice Hall.

Jain AK, Murty MN, and Flynn PJ. (1999) Data clustering: A review. *ACM Comput. Surveys*, 31, 3: 264-323.

Jain AN, Tokuyasu TA, Snijders AM, Segraves R, Albertson DG, and Pinkel D. (2002) Fully automatic quantification of microarray image data. *Genome Res.* 12:325-332.

Jin W, Riley RM, Wolfinger RD, White KP, Passador-Gurgel G, and Gibson G. (2001) The contribution of sex, genotype and age to transcriptional variance in Drosophila melanogaster. *Nature Genetics* 29:389-395.

Jenssen T, Langaas M, Kuo WP, Smith-Sorensen B, Myklebost O, and Hovig E. (2002) Analysis of repeatability in spotted cDNA microarrays. *Nucleic Acids Res.* 30:3235-3244.

Johnson RA, and Wichern DW. (1999) *Applied Multivariate Statistical Analysis.* 4th Ed. Upper Saddle River NJ: Prentice-Hall.

Kepler T, Crosby L, Morgan K. (2000) Normalization and analysis of DNA microarray data by self consistency and local regression. Genome Biol. 3(7):research 0037.1-0037.12.

Kerr MK and Churchill GA. (2001a) Statistical design and the analysis of gene expression microarray data. *Genet. Res.* 77:123 123-128.

Kerr MK and Churchill GA. (2001b) Bootstrapping cluster analysis: Assessing the reliability of conclusions from microarray experiments. *Proc. Nat. Acad. Sci. USA* 98: 8961-8965.

Khan, J, Simon R, Bittner M, Chen Y, Leignton SB, Pohida T, Smith PD, Jiang Y, Gooden GC, Trent JM and Meltzer PS. (1998) Gene expression profiling of alveolar rhabdomyosarcoma with cDNA microarrays. *Cancer Res.* 58: 5009-5013.

Khan J, Wei JS, Ringnér M, Saal LH, Ladanyi M, Westermann F, Berthold F, Schwab M, Antonescu CR, Peterson C, and Meltzer PS. (2001) Classification and diagnostic prediction of cancers using gene expression profiling and artificial neural networks. Nat. Med. 7:673-679.

Kohonen T. (1997) *Self-Organizing Maps.*, Berlin: Springer.

Korn EL, Troendle JF, McShane LM, and Simon, R. (2002) Identifying pre-post chemotherapy differences in gene expression in breast tumours: A statistical method appropriate for this aim. *Brit. J. Cancer 86*: 1093-1096.

Korn EL, Troendle JF, McShane LM, and Simon R. (2003) Controlling the number of false discoveries: Application to high-dimensional genomic data. *J. Stat. Plan. Inference* (in press).

Lachenbruch PA and Mickey MR. (1968) Estimation of error rates in discriminant analysis. *Technometrics* 10:1-11.

Lawless JF. (1982) *Statistical Models and Methods for Lifetime Data.* New York: Wiley.

Lazzeroni, L. and Owen, A. (2002) Plaid models for gene expression data. *Stat. Sinica*, 12(1): 61-86.

Lee C-K, Klopp RG, Weindruch R, and Prolla TA. (1999) Gene expression profile of aging and its retardation by caloric restriction. *Science* 285:1390-1393.

Lee M-L, and Whitmore GA. (2002) Power and sample size for DNA microarray studies. *Stat. Med.* 21:3543-3570.

Lee M-L, Kuo FC, Whitmore GA, and Sklar J. (2000) Importance of replication in microarray gene expression studies: Statistical methods and evidence from repetitive cDNA hybridizations. *Proc. Nat. Acad. Sci. USA* 97: 9831-9839.

Lehmann EL and Stein C. (1949). On the theory of some non-parametric hypotheses. *Ann. Math. Stat.* 20: 28-45.

Li C and Wong WH. (2001a) Model-based analysis of oligonucleotide arrays: Expression index computation and outlier detection. *Proc. Nat. Acad. Sci. USA* 98, 31-36.

Li C and Wong WH. (2001b) Model-based analysis of oligonucleotide arrays: Model validation, design issues and standard error application. *Genome Biol.* 2: 1-11.

Li L, Darden TA, Weinberg CR, Levine AJ, and Pedersen LG. (2001) Gene assessment and sample classification for gene expression data using a genetic algorithm/k-nearest neighbor method. *Comb. Chem. High Throughput Screen.* 4:727 7-39.

Little RJA and Rubin DB. (2002) *Statistical Analysis with Missing Data.* New York: Wiley.

Lockhart DJ, Dong H, Byrne MC, Follettie MT, Gallow MV, Chee MS, Mittmann M, Wang C, Kobayashi M, Horton H, and Brown EL. (1996)

Expression monitoring by hybridization to high-density oligonucleotide arrays. *Nature Biotech.* 14:1675-1680.

Luo J, Duggan DJ, Chen Y, Sauvageot J, Ewing CM, Bittner ML, Trent JM, and Isaacs WB. (2001) Human prostate cancer and benign prostatic hyperplasia: Molecular dissection by gene expression profiling. *Cancer Res.* 61, 4683-4688.

MacDonald TJ, Brown KM, LaFleur B, Peterson K, Lawlor C, Chen Y, Packer RJ, Cogen P, and Stephan DA. (2001) Expression profiling of medulloblastoma: PDGFRA and the RAS/MAPK pathway as therapeutic targets for metastatic disease. Nat Genet 2001; 29:143-152.

MacQueen J. (1967) Some methods for classification and analysis of multivariate observations. In *Proceedings of the Fifth Berkeley Symposium on Mathematical Statistics and Probability*, 1:281-297.

Marubini E and Valsecchi MG. (1995) *Analysing Survival Data from Clinical Trials and Observational Studies*. New York: Wiley.

McShane LM, Radmacher MD, Freidlin B, Yu R., Li M, and Simon R. (2002) Methods for assessing reproducibility of clustering patterns observed in analyses of microarray data. *Bioinf.* 18:1462-1469.

Miller RA, Galecki A, and Shmookler-Reis RJ. (2001) Interpretation, design, and analysis of gene array expression experiments. *J. Gerontol.* 56A: B52-B57.

Milligan GW and Cooper MC. (1985) An examination of procedures for determining the number of clusters in a data set. *Psychometrika*, 50, 159-179.

Naef F, Lim DA, Patil N, and Magnasco MO. (2001) From features to expression: High density oligonucleotide array analysis revisited. LANL e-print physics/0102010.

Newton MA, Kendziorski CM, Richmond CS, Blattner FR, and Tsui KW. (2001) J. Compt. Biol. 8: 37-52.

Nguyen DV and Rocke DM. (2002) Tumor classification by partial least squares using microarray gene expression data. Bioinf. 18:39-50.

Pan W, Lin J, and Le CT. (2002) How many replicates of arrays are required to detect gene expression changes in microarray experiments? A mixture model approach. *Genome Biol.* 3,5 :research 0022.1-0022.10.

Pease AC, Solas D, Sullivan EJ, Cronin MT, Holmes CP, and Fodor SPA. (1994) Light-generated oligonucleotide arrays for rapid DNA sequence analysis. *Proc. Nat. Acad. Sci.* USA 91:5022-5026.

Perou CM, Sorlie T, Eisen MB, van de Rijn M, Jeffrey SS, Rees CA, Pollack JR, Ross DT, Johnsen H, Akslen LA, Fluge O, Pergamenschikov A, Williams C, Zhu SX, Lonning PE, Borresen –Dale AL, Brown PO, and Botstein D. (2000) *Molecular* portraits of human breast tumours. *Nature* 406, 747-752.

Radmacher MD, McShane LM, and Simon R. (2002) A paradigm for class prediction using gene expression profiles. *J. Comput. Biol.* 9:505-511.

Rahnenfuehrer J. (2002) Efficient clustering methods for tumor classification with microarrays. In *Proceedings of the 26th Annual Conference of the Gesellschaft für Klassifikation (GfKl)*, July 22-24, Mannheim, Germany.

Rand WM. (1971) Objective criteria for evaluating clustering methods. *J. Am. Stat. Assoc.* 66: 846-850.

Ripley BD. (1996) *Pattern Recognition and Neural Networks*. Cambridge UK: Cambridge University Press.

Rosenwald A, Wright G, Chan W C, Connors J M, Campo E, Fisher R I, Gascoyne R D, Muller-Hermelink H K, Smeland E B, Giltnane J M, Hurt E M, Zhao H, Averett L, Yang L, Wilson W H, Jaffe E S, Simon R, Klausner RD, Powell J, Duffey PL, Longo DL, Greiner TC, Weisenburger DD, Sanger WG, Dave BJ, Lynch JC, Vose J, Armitage JO, Montserrat E, López-Guillermo A, Grogan TM, Miller TP, LeBlanc M, Ott G, Kvaloy S, Delabie J, Holte H, Krajci P, Stokke T. and Staudt LM (2002) The lymphoma/leukemia molecular profiling project. The use of molecular profiling to predict survival after chemotherapy for diffuse large-B-cell lymphoma. *N. Engl. J. Med.* 346:1937-1947.

Ross DT, Scherf U, Eisen MB, Perou CM, Spellman P, Iyer V, Jeffrey SS, Van de Rijn M, Waltham M, Pergamenschikov A, Lee JCF, Lashkari D, Shalon D, Myers TG, Weinstein JN, Botstein D, and Brown PO. (2000) Systematic variation in gene expression patterns in human cancer cell lines. *Nat. Genet.* 24:227-234.

Schadt EE, Li C, Ellis B, and Wong WH. (2001) Feature extraction and normalization algorithms for high-density oligonucleotide gene expression array data. *J. Cell. Biochem.* Supplement 37:120-125.

Schadt EE, Li C, Su C, and Wong WH. (2000) Analyzing high-density oligonucleotide gene expression array data. *J.Cell. Biochem.* 80:192-202.

Schena M et al. (2000). *Microarray Biochip Technology*. Natick, MA: Eaton.

Schena M, Shalon D, Davis RW, and Brown PO. (1995) Quantitative monitoring of gene expression patterns with a complementary DNA microarray, *Science* 270:467-470.

Sela M, White FH, and Anfinsen CB. (1957) Reductive cleavage of disulfide bridges in ribonuclease. *Science* 125:691-692.

Simon R and Lam A. (2003) BRB-ArrayTools 3.0 User's Guide, http://linus.nci.nih.gov/~brb.

Simon R, Radmacher MD, and Dobbin K. (2002) Design of studies using DNA microarrays. *Genet. Epidem.* 23:21-36.

Simon R, Radmacher MD, Dobbin K, and McShane LM (2003). Pitfalls in the analysis of DNA microarray data for diagnostic and prognostic classification. *J. Nat. Cancer Inst.* 95:14-18.

Snedecor GW and Cochran WG. (1989) *Statistical Methods*, 8th Ed. Ames, IA: Iowa State University Press.

Soille P. (1999) *Morphological Image Analysis: Principles and Applications.* New York: Springer.

Spellman PT, Sherlock G, Zhang MQ, Iyer VR, Anders K, Eisen MB, Brown PO, Botstein D, and Futcher B. (1998) Comprehensive identification of cell cycle-regulated genes of the yeast *saccharomyces cerevisiae* by microarray hybridization. *Molec. Biol.Cell.* 9:3273-3297.

Tamayo P, Slonim D, Mesirov J, Zhu Q, Kitareewan S, Dmitrovsky E, Lander E, and Golub TR. (1999) Interpreting patterns of gene expression with self-organizing maps: Methods and application to hematopoietic differentiation. *Proc. Nat. Acad. Sci. USA* 96, 2907-2912.

Tibshirani, R, Walther, G, and Hastie, T. (2001) Estimating the number of clusters in a data set via the gap statistic. *J. Roy. Stat. Soc., Ser. B, Methodol.* 63 (2), 411-423.

Troyanskaya O, Cantor M, Sherlock G, Brown P, Hastie T, Tibshirani R, Botstein D, and Altman RB. (2001) Missing value estimation methods for DNA microarrays. *Bioinf.* 17: 520-525.

Tseng GC, Oh M, Rohlin L, Lian JC and Wong WH. (2001) Issues in cDNA microarray analysis: Quality filtering, channel normalization, models of variations and assessment of gene effects. *Nucleic Acids Res.* 29: 2549-2557.

Tukey JW. (1993) Tightening the clinical trial. *Controll. Clin. Trials* 14: 266-285.

Tusher VG, Tibshirani R, and Chu G. (2001) Significance analysis of microarrays applied to ionizing radiation response. *Proc. Nat. Acad. Sci. USA* 98: 5116-5121.

Vapnik V. (1998) *Statistical Learning Theory.* New York: Wiley.

Wang X, Ghosh S, and Guo SW. (2001) Quantitative quality control in microarray image processing and data acquisition. *Nucleic Acids Res.* 29, 15:e75.

Wang Y, Lu J, Lee R, Gu Z, and Clark R. (2002) Iterative normalization of cDNA microarray data. *IEEE Tran. Inf. Technol. Biomed.* 6:29-37.

Ward JH. Jr. (1963) Hierarchical grouping to optimize an objective function. *J. Am. Stat. Assoc.* 58: 236-244.

Watson JD, Hopkins NH, Roberts JW, Steitz JA, and Weiner AM. (1987) *Molecular Biology of the Gene*, 4 Ed. Menlo Park CA: Benjamin/Cummings.

West M, Blanchette C, Dressman H, Huang E, Ishida S, Spang R, Zuzan H, Olson JA, Marks JR, and Nevins JR. (2001) Predicting the clinical status of human breast cancer by using gene expression profiles. *Proc Nat. Acad. Sci. USA* 98:11462-11467.

Westfall PH and Young SS. (1993) Resampling-Based Multiple Testing. New York: Wiley.

Wichern DW and Johnson RA. (2002) *Applied Multivariate Statistical Analysis*, 5th Ed., Upper Saddle River, NJ: Prentice-Hall.

Wolfinger RD, Gibson G, Wolfinger ED, Bennett L, Hamadeh H, Bushel P, Afshari C, and Paules RS. (2001) Assessing gene significance from cDNA microarray expression data via mixed models. *J. Comput. Biol.* 8:625-638.

Wright G and Simon R. (2003) Randomized variance hierarchical models for class comparison of in DNA microarray studies. *Bioinf.* (in press).

Xing EP and Karp RM. (2001) CLIFF: Clustering of high-dimensional microarray data via iterative feature filtering using normalized cuts. *Bioinf.* 17 Supplement 1: S306-S315.

Yang YH, and Speed T. Design issues for cDNA microarray experiments. (2002b) *Nature Rev.- Genet.* 3:579-588.

Yang YH, Buckley MJ, Dudoit S, and Speed TP. (2002c) Comparison of methods for image analysis on cDNA microarray data. *J. Comput. Graph. Stat.* 11:108-136.

Yang YH, Buckley MJ, Dudoit S, and Speed TP. (2001) Analysis of cDNA microarray images. *Brief. Bioinf.* 2:341-349.

Yang YH. Dudoit S, Luu P, Lin DM, Peng V, Ngai J, and Speed TP. (2002a) Normalization for cDNA microarray data: a robust composite method addressing single and multiple slide systematic variation. *Nucleic Acids Res.* 30, 4:e15.

Yeung KY, Fraley C, Mutua A, Raftery AE, and Ruzzo WL. (2001a) Model-based clustering and data transformations for gene expression data. *Bioinf.* 17: 977-987.

Yeung, KY, Haynor, D.R., and Ruzzo, W.L. (2001b) Validating clustering for gene expression data. *Bioinf.* 17: 309-318.

Zhang H, Yu C-Y, Singer B, and Xiong M. (2001) Recursive partitioning for tumor classification with gene expression microarray data. *Proc. Nat. Acad. Sci. USA* 2001; 98:6730-6735.

Index

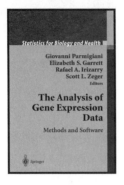
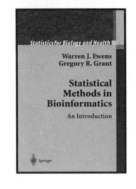
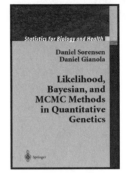